INDEPENDENCE

MEANS

SWIM OR SINK

BY

NEIL B. KIMERER, M.D.

SAGACITY PRESS
Oklahoma City, Ok 73107

BUT

THERE ARE ALL THOSE

CREEPIE CRAWLIES

IN

THE WATER

COPYRIGHT 1995   SAGACITY PRESS
NEIL B. KIMERER, M.D.   1918 -
ALL RIGHTS RESERVED
Manufactured in United States of America
Library of Congress Catalogue   No .95-71246
ISBN No. 0-9648589-1-6

0 9 8 7 6 5 4 3 2 1

TABLE OF CONTENTS

v	Introduction
vii	Foreword
1	Expectations
2	The Differences Between Professionals
3	Credentials
4	Therapist Expectations
5	Thinking and Action
6	Reality
7	Methods
8	Technique
9	Content
10	Touch
11	Struggle
12	Physiological Levels
13	Duration
14	Payment
15	Social Encounters
16	Completion
17	Results

DEDICATION

to

All Those People Who Came
to
Study Themselves
in order
To Achieve a Better Life

INTRODUCTION

Dr. Neil B. Kimerer has been a respected practitioner of psychiatry in Oklahoma City for more than forty years. A graduate of the University of Chicago School of Medicine, he was trained in psychiatry at the famed Menninger Clinic in Topeka, Kansas, and in psychoanalysis as well. After many years of teaching clinical psychiatry at the University of Oklahoma School of Medicine he was named Clinical Professor Emeritus in 1985.

There are few colleagues still in practice who could match the breadth of Dr. Kimerer's experience with psychiatric patients and their families. This book is mainly directed to such people, although there are commentaries on a variety of topical matters relevant to the field of mental health. The result is a vivid narrative that combines practical advice with reflections on issues ranging from professional techniques to public policy and the state of society.

Because the narrative is delivered in Dr. Kimerer's unvarnished and straightforward style, the reader experiences something like a prolonged visit with a veteran practitioner who tells it as he sees it, and has lived it in language that is sometimes gentle, sometimes pedagogic, sometimes acerbic, but always unmistakenly the author's own.

Here then, is an intensely personal distillation of a lifetime's experience of work in the field of psychiatry. One comes away with an unusual sense of knowing the author, because he expresses himself without apology, in plain language, and with utmost candor. This is clearly the voice of a man who takes his profession seriously, who cares deeply about his patients, and who sometimes despairs that our society does not yet fulfill all of it's responsibilities. Whether or not one agrees with everything

Neil Kimerer has to say, one must admire his dedication, his passion, and in giving of himself as he does in this book- his generosity.

> Louis Jolyon West, M.D.
> Professor of Psychiatry
> UCLA School of Medicine

FOREWORD

For the past four decades the flood of pressure coming from organized psychiatry and its influence on the congress to supply mental health to every citizen through legislation, massive expenditure has reached a point of no return. It has not improved the mental health of the public nor has it provided adequate care to those who seek to use the services.

One gets the impression that what it has done is empty the state hospitals and transferred those populations to an explosive expansion of nursing homes and what are euphemistically called Comprehensive Mental Health Centers, Mental Health Clinics or Counseling Centers. It has also helped to create a massive debt for the nation through deficit financing. Congress has made promises which have led the public to abdicate its sense of responsibility to and for itself. The creation of this gigantic system has created chaos in the mental health "industry". For the past four decades the federal platform of deficit spending has supported massive waste, greed and fraud throughout the nation and has created a bureaucracy which is not necessary. It is by this means that the members of congress have succeeded in maintaining themselves by being reelected 98% of the time. The congress has bought votes with all forms of deficit spending..

Furthermore, in terms of the professions of medicine and mental health it has denigrated those professionals who feel a responsibility toward the people who they see and has substituted mediocre services at tremendous expense.

Now we are in a period of retraction and retrenching because of the costs and the medical profession is getting the blame for costs of all medical expense, medicare, medicaid, disability and every service related to the delivery of medical care. The congress has maintained itself by deficit spending and has expanded all federal programs to a point at which the individuals who receive those funds now feel that they are "entitled" to them and have lost the capacity to fend for themselves. The congress has told them that they cannot fend for themselves and has encouraged them to become dependent on the public deficit spending largesse.

The business of the 'entitlement' programs has become a way of life for the entire nation since the election of Franklin Delano Roosevelt and the instigation of social security over fifty years ago.

All of the subsidy programs for industry, such as farming, housing, and a myriad of others, other than the traditional ones of maintaining communications, supervising transportation facilities, conducting foreign relations, and maintaining our international posture in military requirements against the potential threat of either attack or invasion by foreign powers. Few of such Federal services have done the job they were intended to do. The government has now expanded itself to promise "cradle to the grave" care for the people far beyond the expectations of socialists, such as Norman Thomas, who have repeatedly lost elections.

With this as a back drop, what is happening in mental health has led me to the consideration of putting together what I know about what is happening in Mental Health.

It disturbs me a great deal that a significant fraction of the public no longer feels that it is responsible for its own livelihood or that it is responsible for its own sustenance. At the same time the massive outlays for the control of drug habits and control of crime have not attained their idealistically promised goals. The judiciary has now become so lax and legislative in its application of the principles on which this country was founded (Bork, Robert) that the original system is grossly distorted and is being destroyed.

The "Annonimiti" of various government, corporate, associations of corporations, civil servants, bureaucrats, regulators, third party payers, reviewers, supervisors, etc., border on being specialized secret agents because their names are not known to those who they oversee and control, yet they cannot be personally held responsible to account for their decisions, and fiats. Still, they have the power to inflict civil, and sometimes, criminal punishment by imposing sanctions, fines, and incarceration "for the good of society in accordance with law". They have the authority to impose their will on the people performing the service by changing the regulations, which have the force of law, at their personal discretion and without representation of the public.

We are reaching a point of no return unless something is done to halt this trend and for the public to educate itself in order to compete that individuals may supply their own needs. The facilities, books, and libraries already exist but what is missing is the drive to care for oneself. Students, parents and institutions turn to the giant Washington Mismanagement Team to take care of them.

If there is any hope for this country something has to be done soon. There has to he a heart rending, belt tightening in individuals who live here to get along on what they can personally produce.

We who live here are blessed with the providence, natural resources, opportunities and with what once was a constitution, created with the foresight of our founding organizers of this government to strive toward individual responsibility. At that time there was only individual responsibility and very little government. What government there was became the thorn to stimulate the American

Revolution and create the government of the people, for the people and by the people.

Unless we regain that devotion to individual responsibility, freedom in this nation will very shortly be a thing of the past. Society does not create criminals. Individual lack of personal responsibility creates criminals.

It is my intention to inform the public what the circumstances are should they seek a change in mental health for themselves.

I thank all those people who have helped me over the years in providing me a living and, hopefully, I have been of some positive service to them as they were able to investigate themselves or with medication get calmed down to a point where they could manage their own lives as is necessary for each of us. I have not treated anybody. I am unable to change anybody. Hopefully what I have done is assist them in their finding their own way to a more satisfactory lifestyle than they had before they came to me.

The question arises, how do you teach, or "give" the opportunity for the people of the country to make the hard decisions that are necessary and the deprivation which may be necessary for them to become "self sufficient" again. It is a natural state during their lifetimes to be exposed to the vicissitudes of the uncertainty of not knowing what will be ahead for them in the future. The kind of false dependency that has been instilled in the public in this country for the past, now almost three generations, is such that it is seeking security; seeking evenness; and in the newspaper this morning it is seeking guarantees for income without work, if possible, at someone else's expense of energy.

Unfortunately, nature does not give guarantees. We are all subject to its vicissitudes and it remains the strongest force in existence surpassing all of the nuclear weapons which have been developed.

But to give up those guarantees and to live on what one is able to accomplish for oneself is a major undertaking. It is not something which can be decreed from Washington by law, except by rescinding many of the current guarantees which exist and in particular, by rescinding the funding.

In writing the laws during the last fifty years the congress has been so self serving that it has not had sufficient statesmanship, individually and collectively, to consider what and how its actions today will impact the nature of the country a hundred or two hundred years from now, particularly in the aspect of what the attitude and lifestyle of the people will be in terms of their being able to care for themselves.

It is necessary to look over the ends of our noses in order to see the horizon or surely we will be seeing the sunset of individual responsibility if the present trend continues.

The pronouns "he", "his", and "him", as used at various points in this book, are not intended to convey the masculine gender alone; this usage is employed in a generic sense so as to avoid awkward grammatical constructions which would likely occur due to the limitations of the English language.

Bork, Robert H. The Tempting of America
   The Free Press, N.Y. 1990 ISBN 0-02-903761-1

CHAPTER 1

At some time or another in our lives most of us would like the world to treat us better- or so we think. At least we would like to have things going our way better than we think we have now.

Sometimes we feel so jittery we think we will jump out of our skin- or we feel like little springs are underneath our skin and shimmering, all at the same time. If we think about getting some relief; that relief seems impossible to attain or to find before we fall apart in a heap or pool of flesh and blood. Nothing seems to relieve the tension and we sometimes wish we could explode and get it over with if it would give some relief. Finally, in desperation, you try to get some help to relieve the tension.

If you go voluntarily to a therapist you have a much better chance to get relief than if some one else makes you go. To go voluntarily means that you know that you have a problem of emotional strain, and however severe, there is a better chance of finding some relief if you know you need it.

There are different ways of describing the tensions or maladjustments to living. Some people think of them as emotional problems and some think of them as mental. Often these terms are used interchangeably. Most professionals think of them as emotional and most people, patients, think of them as mental. Most people who go to see a psychiatrist or other professional don't think of themselves as patients, or clients. All they feel is that they are not functioning as well as they want to and want someone to change them so they don't feel the tension. Anything to get some relief.

Furthermore "emotional strain" or "stress" is not always caused by emotions alone. A significant number of people have physical problems which alter their normal emotional functioning and such people need thorough physical, chemical and endocrine evaluations and treatment for whatever imbalances are found before a purely emotional or psychiatric system of treatment is begun. Without a physically healthy body, and mind, it is futile to try to correct what seem to be emotional problems.

We are all different; we are different physically; we are different mentally and those very subtle differences of our body structure, our personalities and our minds is what makes us unique individuals. Each of us is a part of nature's experiment as to of what we are constituted, the way we react and all our physiological and emotional problems. Each of us is born with a different set of genes and the only exception to that statement is identical twins where two people are born from a single ovum and their gene patterns are or should be identical. Even then there may be differences in the way in which life treats them, even in utero. One or the other of them may have had a little more blood delivered to them through the common placenta or the separate placenta and one or the other of them might have different things happen to them just in the process of birth itself, as well as all the other things that happen to them after they are born. So that in a sense no two people, even identical twins, are identical.

Many people have problems which cannot be corrected. They are born with hormone or metabolism problems which give their body structure and physiology different patterns for existence than they want. They have no choice but to live with what they were given at birth even though some of those problems may not appear until they are in their teens or older. That doesn't mean that they are "sick" physically but rather that the conditions of their existence are dictated by the shapes or sizes their body structure or by the genes they inherited which dictate their physiological processes. They don't have to like what they were given but they can't change their particular conditions of existence. Many of them feel miserable and frustrated because they can't change - like the proverbial fish out of water. They may feel themselves to be undesirable, unwanted, unloved, awkward, and out of place.

There are many minor and major physical illnesses which can alter one's adjustment to life. Sometimes what appears to be a "mental" problem can disappear when a physical problem is corrected. Thyroid malfunctions, for example directly influence other hormonal systems in the body. The chronic ache and pain of peptic ulcers, muscle soreness, electrolyte imbalances, diabetes, poor liver function, alcoholism, hormone imbalances, and various diseases of the blood all have greater influence than just in their own organ system. The use of "mind expanding" drugs can permanently change the physiology of the central nervous system if it goes beyond the tolerance for that particular person and no one has enough knowledge to determine exactly what that tolerance is. All and any of such deviations can alter the manner in which the central nervous system works and can seem to be a "mental" or "neurotic" problem. Insomnia is a frequent complaint which can accompany any imbalance and be enough in itself to seek help. Heart problems may lead to insufficient blood going to the brain to keep you alert or to keep you awake, or awaken you. It isn't necessary for you to have pain to feel that "something is wrong" but be unable to be any more specific than that when you tell the doctor. Difficulty breathing can also cause what appears to be fear and anxiety - or depression. Sometimes tumors, without pain, can press on some organ to give you the feeling that some thing is wrong and create panic or anxiety. There are limitless possibilities of organ malfunction which can affect your adjustment and create your symptoms, not just emotions. Don't forget that emotions are, themselves, complex physiological and hormonal functions.

Also, worry about any physical problem may cause more distress than the physical problem itself. In which instance the person is subject to a double whammy: the physical problem and the emotional problem of the worry. In such a circumstance the first step is to reduce the anxiety (worry) to useful levels rather than disruptive ones and that may take some effort to accomplish. Sometimes when that is accomplished there is little need to spend a lot of time on the physical problem, and it can be treated much more effectively to the extent it can be treated. To divide one's energies between worry and treatment of physical problems may leave too little energy to modify the physical problems. When the emotional problems are under some control then treatment of the physical problems becomes much easier and more effective within the scope of treatment which is possible. The converse is also true. Successful treatment of a physical problem may obliterate an "emotional" problem. The opposite of what I have just stated is also true, that is, that many physical problems in and of themselves can cause alterations of the physiology of the central nervous system and what appears to be an anxiety is actually a direct manifestation of those physical problems.

Whatever those physical problems may be they may be mediated by hormones or by different alterations of physiology as a result of nutritional alterations, excesses or deficiencies. They may be alterations of physiology as a result of an inability of that particular organ to function as most organs function in other people. There may be any and all kinds of variations of disease to create the problems which may be manifested as mental or emotional ones.

Some fat people are fat because of their genetics or hormone imbalances, not because they eat too much. They may need psychotherapy to help adjust to a set of circumstances over which they have no control and to learn to live with their limitations but not to blame themselves because they are overweight. When they can tackle their problem of being overweight directly and with less emotional tension about it they have a much better chance of setting themselves on a path of self control to better control their weight. When they can realistically accept the fact that their genes are the cause of their problems, and give up the unrealistic ideal of being like the trimmest movie star when that is not possible for them, their lives will be much more calm and peaceful. It takes a great deal of self knowledge and acceptance to give up those unrealistic ideals and goals. I, at one time, had a resident in psychiatry from Mexico who told me that the United States of America is the only nation in the world where people who live in poverty have to go on a diet to lose weight.

Just think of what a horrible disaster it would be if we did have some control over our genes. If we had control over our genes then we would be able to change ourselves to whatever preconceived notion we have, or we might have, of what we think we would like to be like. If we were given only one set of change we could make, how would we be able to decide what would be the best way for us to change? I don't think anybody would be able to really understand or project all the possibilities of eventualities which could occur if we did change our genes.

I think it is very fortunate that we are not able to control our genes. What is unfortunate is the fact that we still long, often, to try to make ourselves over into what we think we would like to be. Without actually being able to know what it would be like to be what we think we would like to be.

There are people who, through the process of birth, have misshapen limbs, or some parts of their bodies which are not in the same proportions as most people. These people, too, must make an adjustment to their bodies. To them, their shape or proportion is all they have ever known and they don't feel different from anyone else but to those who do not have such changes they may look "funny" and stare or make remarks that indicate that the difference had been noticed. Some crude people may even make unkind remarks and demonstrate their own lack of adaptability and consideration. There are other people who may have been injured and left with some distortion of their appearance - such as burns, twisted limbs from broken bones, or defects left from necessary surgery to correct an injury, infection or illness. Such unlucky ones have to learn to live with the changes which are thrust upon them and that might require a lot of emotional readjustment. They will have their changed appearance all the rest of their lives, but they don't have to like it even though they are forced to live with it.

Every person who seeks help does so under strained circumstances. To some people the fact that they are seeking help marks the end of a period of self examination which may have gone on for years. Going to see a psychiatrist for the first time is always a very emotionally painful step and fraught with anxiety. While going through that door into the office the question "What am I doing here?" goes through your head. " Maybe I can back out of it" may be the next thought. Then you sit down and the psychiatrist tries to be affable and to help you to feel a little more comfortable. You find yourself with your emotional nakedness hanging out for all to see. Then the talk begins and some of the fear is eased - just a little. But it is a long way from being abolished or relieved to any significant extent.

There are also those who have such desperation to get relief from their tensions that they dump themselves on the professional and sit there waiting for the magic words to clear away all the anger, terrors, fears, insomnia, bad dreams, anxiety or despondency. Such people are just as certain to be disappointed as are those who expect all the fears and tensions to evaporate. No magic words issue forth and help seems too far away to do any good, and too late to be of any use.

If you go voluntarily you may leave that first interview wondering why you went and what you received during the time you spent, for a lot of money. Hopefully, you may feel a little relieved and not feel so tense about returning.

Sometimes the person is forced into seeking change by some authority outside themselves, such as the family, various social authorities, police, sheriff, or court. This book is not about you, nor for you if such circumstances take you to the therapist. If it is necessary that some one else forces you to seek the aid of a psychiatrist or other counselor, the likelihood of that treatment being successful is very small. You will probably not cooperate to any significant degree although you may seem placid on the surface - that part of you which you want the world to see but underneath that masking surface is more likely to be an attitude of "make me" which automatically defeats the purpose for which you are sent. With that kind of a defiant encounter nothing the therapist can say or do is likely to loosen your hold on your preconceived notions and fear of other people, regardless how the therapist relates to you. The therapist has a tough job of trying to get you to loosen your hold on your preconceived notions that all the people in the world are to be feared. It is true that there are people in the world who should be feared, but there are also people in the world who you can trust. The secret in getting along well is to be able to tell the difference and be afraid of those who are to be feared and be trusting of those who can be trusted. That's what we ought to learn in the process of growing up but unfortunately most people have not grown up completely and hang on to a lot of preconceived wrong notions.

The entire process of treatment is getting to know yourself differently than you knew yourself at the time you first went for treatment. There is no magic way of changing. Remember that what you have to work with to change yourself is the mass of wrong notions and the way in which you communicate those wrong notions. You have to use an adjustment system which doesn't work well to find an adjustment system which works better. The poorly working adjustment system is all you have at the time you go for help and it will be necessary for you to listen to the therapist even though you don't want to hear what he has to say at the same time you want to be different. If someone, or social agency, made you go in the first place and you didn't want to go the situation is even harder to adjust to and you wont want to adjust. Therapists are people - no more - and hopefully, no less. They react to you the same as they would react to anybody else, if they are honest with themselves. Psychiatric, social or counseling theory is for the benefit of easing the tension of the therapist - to give the therapist the assurance that he knows what he is doing in "treatment". Theory doesn't benefit you, the patient, directly and what theory the "professional" thinks he is practicing doesn't mean that that's what you get out of it, nor that is what is going on during the therapy.

Most people who come to a professional's office want their anxieties, sleeplessness, insomnia, lethargy, despondency, or whatever problem bothers them cured with one visit. It would be miraculous if that could be so. Patients usually don't care how that goal is accomplished - except for tales of unhappy experiences they might have received from someone else who had had some treatment. However, had the tales included moral values being infringed, or sexual advances made, the difficulty they have coming in to see a therapist themselves is greatly increased. In my view no therapist has the right to infringe your moral values.

Just as some people want to be cured in a single session so they want to be cured with a single dose or day of medications. Medications do not work that fast. They, too, need time to work and the physician cannot speed up those processes in the body which takes in the medications and distributes them in usable form to those organs on which they work. Sometimes it is necessary for the body to be "saturated" with the medications before the medications take effect and that process may take as long as three or four weeks. After that, the effectiveness of the medications may take several months to change your personality, sensations or physiology in the central nervous system. So you are bound to be disappointed when after the first or second dose nothing has happened. It hasn't happened to the extent you can see or feel the result you want. Further, it may take the medications several more days to have the effect which they can create, and even that is not an instantaneous process but rather a gradual one. Sometimes the dose of medications is not enough to alter your feeling regardless of how long you take them. That same medication may be a perfectly good one at a different dose level. It takes time and patience to find the proper dosage level for any particular person and the physician is as helpless as you are to alter that process.

People are different. What medicine works for one person may never work for another. So changes on a trial and error basis may need to be made until the medication which works for you is found. Further, some people react with "side" effects which are not desirable and which do not occur in other people, in which case it is necessary to change to a new medication. Also some medications have temporary undesirable effects which will go away if that drug is taken for a few days more and then it may become effective without the discomfort. Sometimes no known medication will give relief. Patience is a virtue of which most emotionally disturbed people have little; you are already very uncomfortable and any added discomfort, even temporary, may make your life seem less tolerable and more frantic. Meanwhile, the physician is doing his best to relieve you of your tensions even though it may not seem so to you.

Some medications work faster than others, depending on what the patient needs to alleviate his symptoms. Physicians don't have any more magic medications than they have magic words - which are none. Medications are always either a necessity or a compromise. Sometimes in order to hold us together so we can talk, the psychiatrist offers a prescription. Some psychiatrists rely on prescriptions to do all the work, but most of the time, even when the medications are effective without undesirable side effects, what you do with yourself to unravel the onset and reaction patterns you have developed to reach such a sad state is the crucial test. If you can't do that for one reason or another - primarily because you are too afraid of what you might find out about yourself - then you may have to settle for the medications and be grateful for them.

Some people (a great many of them) have never examined themselves emotionally and mentally and don't know how to proceed. They look to the therapist for a cook book method to get to the bottom of themselves with little or no effort on their part. So they too will be disappointed, and perhaps angry that they can't get the "answers" they want - without effort. They also don't know how to make the effort and feel uncomfortable in dealing with the feeling which comes out, or doesn't come out. You may be embarrassed if the feelings let go with a rush and the tears start flowing, or anger spouts by blowing off verbal steam with no provocation. The embarrassment when that happens may give you the feeling of wanting to crawl under the carpet to hide in shame. The psychiatrist should take it in stride and try to help you accept such unprovoked feelings with as gentle an attitude as you can accept - and without recrimination or fear of you. Psychotherapy is an emotional experience of living and when it is effective can help you make much better adjustments in the future but no one - especially not your therapist, can plan a course of psychotherapy with predetermined steps and predetermined intervals or numbers of appointments. It is a sharing of life's experience in the office with the psychiatrist which is the treatment. The psychiatrist must also share that life's experience with you or there can be no therapy. It is not a one way street - for you only.

You might expect the psychiatrist to wield his magic and talking to you to tell you how to manage yourself without you having to tell him very much about yourself. You may want all the answers; THE answer in a few words so you can get on with your life, cured and forever placid and different, or at least much better able to cope with life. The only real answer is that there is no single secret answer. Treatment is a mutual experience. Psychiatrists don't cure you - you do- with the psychiatrist's assistance. Almost everybody expects that the psychiatrist will provide all the right words, advice, or directions for better behavior, or the right medicine, to relieve them of their anxieties and tensions. Psychiatrists can not read minds.

All such treatment whether with medicine or not, is a mutual experience and interchange of emotions so that both may gather information to make new adjustments to the new situation and also to improve your capacity to make adjustments to the uncertain and unpredictable future. Before you are finished you will know the therapist as well as he will know you and you should be on equal footing.

Such changes take a long time. Perhaps more time than you planned for, or would like to take. There are no short cuts to permanent change in attitude or behavior whether through medication or what is euphemistically called psychotherapy. You have only that adjustment with which you go into treatment to apply to treatment and try to change. As you proceed to learn more about yourself and are able to make small adjustments, the process seems to become easier and your expectations of major, or quick change in yourself, also become more realistic and you learn to live with the new you. Very small changes in attitude and behavior can make a major difference in your life as you go through it but you can learn as you do change and then the old you seems to get lost in memory and may seem like a bad dream, almost unbelievable. It will seem incredible to you that you used to be like you were, if you remember it at all. If you do remember the old life, it will be much more empty of all the forceful emotions which you had before treatment. But the feelings will be there, just not so dominating and consuming.

The problem of relating to a psychiatrist comes when expectations are so powerful and dominating that you are not able to face reality, but see all of what is happening to you as so disastrous that your life seems empty and with no future. Then is the time to somehow take a look at yourself and ask: "How much am I expecting? How much am I contributing to this mess I am in? I am responsible for myself and the messes I find myself in whether I like it or not. Whether I made the mess or not, only I can get myself out."

If I want to be whole and self sufficient, Independence means Swim or Sink. Swim!

Bork, Robert H. <u>The Tempting of America</u>
Free Press, N.Y. 1990 ISBN 0-02-903761-1

CHAPTER 2

Most people who seek help for their "nerves" have no knowledge about the education to which the professional they consult is exposed. They come to a "Doctor" and most think that a psychiatrist is a kind of doctor different from a Doctor of Medicine. They do not know the difference between a Psychiatrist (M.D.) and a Psychologist (Ph.D. or D.Psy) or any other type of Ph.D. They are more confused if someone with a Th.D. (Doctor of Theology) or an L.L.D. (Doctor of Letters) or D.Ed. (Doctor of Education) does counseling and is called "Doctor", to which they are entitled. Currently lawyers are awarded a J.D. degree (Juris Doctor) by many law schools and they, too, should be addressed as "Doctor". So I present the following information for clarification.

ALLOPATHIC PHYSICIAN

In the current practice of medicine practically all physicians are educated as allopathic physicians.

The allopathic means that the physician will use any means which is scientifically demonstrated or reasonable to cure his patient whether it will be medicine, surgery, manipulation, diet, recommendations for a lifestyle of living or anything which in his opinion will be of benefit to make the patient's life and health better.

There are many other types of systems of medicine which have been practiced over the years and most of these are not being practiced to any significant extent at the present time.

One of these is the "Homeopathic Physician". The homeopathic physician practices medicine prescribing medication at a dosage considerably less than the allopathic physician. In the theory of homeopathic medicine it is believed that the prescriptions of medication should be no greater and no stronger than that which is found naturally in the human body and would be in itself therapeutic. Thus "homeo" means "the same" or in balance with nature. The dosages of medications prescribed are minuscule when compared to those dosages used by the allopathic physician. Also, the homeopathic physician strictly limits his medications to those medicaments which occur only in nature, and in the form in which they occur in nature. Some of the medicines were pretty crude - ground root etc.

Another system of medicine which is not now prominent and is in somewhat disrepute is called "Naturopathic Physicians".

In the naturopathic system of medicine it is thought that no substance should be given to a patient in the form of medication which does not occur in nature. No man-made substance should ever be prescribed as a medication as that is foreign to the nature of man.

No surgery is prescribed in naturopathic systems and under these circumstances there are many conditions that do not receive adequate treatment. Nonetheless, in naturopathic system of medicine injuries are also treated because they are a natural occurrence and they are treated without surgery if possible, because surgery is frowned upon and not accepted as a form of treatment because it is not "a natural" way because nature does not provide surgery.

There is one other now out dated system: "Eclectic." The eclectic physician believed that in order to provide the best medicaments possible that it was necessary for him to mix and formulate them himself. Therefor, he bought or grew his own herbs and dried, or extracted the essences of the medications he wished to make and was his own manufacturer and pharmacist of his drugs. He did not limit his pharmacopoeia except to those medications which he could manufacture himself. He also did surgery when indicated.

The practice of medicine has so changed in the past century that my father-in-law graduated from the Eclectic Medical School in Cincinnati, Oh., in 1884 and my wife and I cleaned his one room manufacturing laboratory in his office attached to the home in which my wife was raised when we prepared the house and office for sale in 1944 after I graduated from an Allopathic Medical School. We have the monaural black walnut stethoscope with which he went into practice in 1884.

The most common system of medicine which is now in use other than allopathic system is the osteopathic system of medicine. We will discuss osteopathic physicians and osteopathic systems of medicine later in this chapter.

ALLOPATHIC PSYCHIATRIST

A psychiatrist is an M.D. who has spent the same length of time obtaining his license to practice Medicine as any other physician. He is not required to have graduated from college with a Bachelor's Degree to enter medical school, but 95% of medical school applicants will have a Bachelor's degree at the time of matriculation into medical school, which lasts four years. He has also spent at least four years after graduation from medical school in "post graduate" study, three years of which is the specialized study of psychiatry. This is the same length of time as any other specialist in medicine, general surgery, internal medicine, obstetrics and gynecology, pediatrics, radiology, pathology or other medical specialty. If he is certified by the American Board of Psychiatry and Neurology he has had at least two years of practice of his specialty of psychiatry prior to taking the examination for certification.

The three year period he spends learning to be a specialist in psychiatry is called a residency, as it is called in any other specialty of medicine.

He may or may not have had personal treatment during or after his residency. Personal treatment is not a requirement to become a psychiatrist but sometime in the course of his specialty training and supervision he probably has had some degree of emotional disturbance for which, hopefully, he has received treatment.

In his training he should have been exposed to some experience in Group Therapy, Community Psychiatry, Individual Psychotherapy, Child Psychiatry, Emergency Psychiatry, Psychopharmacology, and Neurology of men and women as well as diseases which affect the body and mind, drugs which affect the body and mind, treatment of medical and psychiatric emergencies as well as an introduction to psychological testing. He should have had personal supervision in both individual and group psychotherapy. Because there are so many theories to which he was exposed his theoretical bias will depend on the training program where he received his training. He should have had a smattering of reading contact with a majority of psychiatric theories and practice. How he practices will be the result of his personality and teaching and will vary from psychiatrist to psychiatrist, the same as with other physicians. Remember, medical school is aimed primarily at treatment of the body and not of the mind. In his residency he spends an amount of time equal to medical school studying the mind. He is the only professional who studies both, body and mind.

We are in an era of anti-medicine even though specialized physicians spend the longest formal education time of any profession, trying to learn and treat the complexities of human lives and behavior. Physicians are not perfect and some do exploit their prestige to the disadvantage of their patients but such are very few of the group- less than three percent as a rule. Nonetheless, that three percent occasionally give the entire profession a poor reputation. Such a small percentage of deviation would make other professions seem perfect indeed - yet in physicians the entire profession is often branded as being untrustworthy and greedy. People and politicians envy and admire the individuality of physicians, at the same time. Some people who envy more than admire are now using their political power to reduce that individuality and mediocratize medical care. Yet, it is that very individuality which has provided the best medical care known to mankind, and the most readily available at the least cost, although not all aspects of current medical delivery are perfect, nor evenly distributed in these United States. Perfection cannot be obtained by legislative fiat, tyrannical decree, committee, regulation, nor appropriation of money. Nor can it be achieved by distributing the physician's multiple functions around to other professions with less comparable education. Psychoanalysis is a specialized form of the practice of psychiatry.

In years past it wasn't necessary for a physician to have had a formal psychiatric residency in order to be enrolled in an institute for learning psychoanalysis and subsequently become a member of the American Psychoanalytic Association or perhaps some other association of psychoanalysts. At one time in the past when the American Psychoanalytic Association attempted to have itself designated, by the Department of Interior of the federal government, the sole educating authority for psychoanalysis. They were refused.

They were refused because they recognized only the training in their own individual institutes and did not accept training in any other institute other than those approved by the American Psychoanalytic Association.

There were some thirty different groups and organizations who practiced forms of psychoanalysis based on slightly different theories with different emphasis on parts of the original psychoanalytic concepts. Such organizations contested the designation of the American Psychoanalytic Association as the sole training authority for the title "psychoanalyst".

Currently psychoanalysis is not being practiced anywhere near as frequently as it was in the past. The reason being that in its primary concepts psychoanalysis rejects the idea of using medication as a form of treatment.

In the recent years however, many psychoanalysts have deviated from their original conservative approach of not using medication and are using medication as an adjunct to psychoanalysis. Whether or not that particular psychoanalyst uses medications will depend solely on his individual concepts.

Also, in the past, all members of the American Psychoanalytic Association were required to be MD's but in recent years the standards for membership in the American Psychoanalytic Association have been modified to include some psychologists and professionals educated in other professions. So, if you go to see a psychoanalyst as your therapist you need to look for some different kinds of evidence of his education and his acceptance in the various psychoanalytic associations. He may or may not be a member of the American Medical Association or the American Psychiatric Association or other psychiatric organizations than his psychoanalytic associations.

Of the types of psychotherapy that are practiced, psychoanalysis has received the most publicity of all the various kinds and types of psychotherapy except for Eric Berne's "Transactional Analysis".

As most everyone knows, psychoanalysis was originated by Sigmund Freud beginning approximately in 1895 and it has achieved a considerable diversity of reputation depending on ones attitude about psychoanalysis in general. It has also had more types of definitions applied to it than any other system of thinking in psychiatry.

Some of the theoretical aspects of psychoanalysis will be included in the body of this book later on, I wanted to bring it up now because it has been only recently that psychoanalysis has been practiced by psychologists as well as physicians. In the United States in order to be a psychoanalyst and to practice as a psychoanalyst, it was necessary for one to be a physician but this is no longer necessarily true. Many forms of "Psychoanalytic Psychotherapy" are rampant. Some of these differences of opinion and definitions of practice will come up later in different chapters.

OSTEOPATHIC PHYSICIANS (D.O.)

Most physicians are MD's educated in the allopathic tradition (to use any method which in the art, skill of science, drugs, surgery, appliances, psychotherapy, etc which are thought to be of use to identify the illness and treat the patient to relieve him of disease). There have been many other systems of medicine practiced in the past, and mostly abandoned by reason of their ineffectiveness. Eclectic and homeopathic were two of the theories of medical practice which have practically vanished. One type of practice continues to flourish although the original concepts of the system were quite deviant from the allopathic system.

In 1892 Dr. Eugene Still began to teach the theory that all of the ailments to which mankind is subject can be explained on the basis of a misalignment of the skeleton. With that as the basic cause of all diseases of mankind, Dr. Still's therapeutic system was to realign the skeleton so all the bones of the skeleton were in their natural association with one another and thereby cure the patient's illness.

With his theory he began teaching and established an Osteopathic School of Medicine at Kirksville, Missouri in 1892 and since then the Osteopathic Physician (D.O.) has become more numerous and prospered.

Over the years the education of the Osteopath has greatly altered and it now includes the same scientific curriculum to which Allopathic physicians are exposed. Much of the curriculum of education for the Osteopathic physician is identical with that of Allopathic physicians.

The original meaning and the original direction in which Dr. Still took his system of medicine has virtually disappeared. Gradually Osteopathic Medicine has adopted many of the forms of treatment of the Allopathic system and currently the practice of medicine and surgery by Doctors of Osteopathy (D.O.) is hardly distinguishable from Allopathic medicine.

Such D.O. and M.D. physicians occasionally intermingle in their professional associations. For the most part the D.O. specialists obtain their specialty training in their own institutions and their professional organizations generally prefer to recognize only that training received in Osteopathic Hospitals, and they recognize only their own professional certification, with some exceptions.

It is now possible for a physician with a D.O. degree to obtain specialty training in the Allopathic hospitals in some specialties. Some state legislatures (Ca.) have authorized the granting of an M.D. degree to those D.O.'s who had applied within a specified time. Many D.O.'s rejected the offer. Many younger ones accepted it and are now counted among the Allopathic Physicians, at least in California.

In psychiatry whether a person holds a D.O. or an M.D. degree is inconsequential, as there were no residencies in psychiatry in Osteopathic hospitals until the past few years. All residencies in Psychiatry were in Allopathic hospitals. Thus, on satisfactory completion of his residency training any D.O. was eligible to take the examination for Certification in Psychiatry or Neurology by the American Board of Psychiatry and Neurology depending on the emphasis of his training. It is a strange turn in the Osteopathic specialties which recognize Osteopathic psychiatrists but few of the professional Osteopathic associations or hospitals offers a residency in psychiatry . Thus any D.O. who offers his services as a psychiatrist either has received specialty training in his own discipline, or he has fulfilled the same requirements for specialized training as have the Allopathic psychiatrists.

In the event that he has received Allopathic Psychiatric training he may be certified by the American Board of Psychiatry and Neurology and may display that certificate as indication that he has received the same education as the Allopathic physician and has passed the same specialty examination. In the event he has not sought certification he will be entitled to display the certificate either of successful completion of his residency, or a letter from the American Board of Psychiatry and Neurology stating his eligibility to be examined for certification, or both. He may also display membership certificates in professional Osteopathic organizations if he is a member of his Osteopathic professional organizations.

PSYCHOLOGIST

The Psychologist usually has a Ph.D. degree (Doctor of Philosophy). He may or may not have specialized in Clinical Psychology. In the past several years a new degree has been established, D.Psy. (Doctor of Psychology) which is what is called a "definitive" degree because it does not require the candidate to do any original psychological research to complete the requirements for the degree. All Ph.D. degrees regardless of their speciality of knowledge require a "dissertation" based on original research in their field of speciality. The D. Psy. makes no such requirement.

There are about thirty seven subspecialties in psychology (from what I could ascertain from the American Psychological Association). Some dissertations I have read in Clinical Psychology related to experimental work with pigeons, fish, or primates and statistics, but not people. The psychologist is not required to study the human body, nor to interrelate bodily functions with mental ones.

He is prohibited from prescribing drugs, although there are some programs which are considering authorizing psychologists to prescribe some types of drugs. Some states are also considering, or have already, permitted psychologists to admit patients to hospitals although when they do so they can only admit with the cooperation of a physician to treat physical ailments. Psychologists are not yet licensed to do physical examinations and therapy of the body. He has never formally studied those functions of people. His studies are not standardized for course material and content and vary from candidate to candidate and from various theories of psychology among universities. He usually spends at least three years obtaining his Ph.D. and after he receives his Doctoral Degree and he may have spent about two years in post Doctoral studies to qualify for his "diplomate" status. An examination for diplomate status may not be required. Few practicing psychologists are diplomates in Clinical Psychology. He likes to be called "Doctor", to which he is entitled - but that does not qualify him to treat people for physical illness. Many states now have laws licensing or certifying the psychologist to practice, but do not necessarily require him to have a degree in clinical psychology, nor a Ph.D., as such requirements vary from state to state. A license to practice psychology usually makes him eligible to do counseling in many fields: Family, Group, Psychological Testing. Vocational Testing, Personality evaluation, Social psychology, Criminology, etc..

He usually avoids calling what he does treatment, or therapy, as those terms are ordinarily reserved for medical treatment although it is very frequent that the psychological examination summary may contain suggestions regarding a more, or most, probable diagnosis. He is usually restricted in making diagnosis of his clients, as diagnostics are usually reserved for physicians. In some medical teaching institutions psychologists are now in positions of making administrative judgment as to the adequacy of psychiatric training when they have never had formal exposure to what they are judging and are prohibited by law from writing prescriptions and doing physical forms of treatment, as well as taking final responsibility for treatment. They sometimes claim to know more about personal adjustment than do psychiatrists and frequently become involved in individual counseling, group counseling, and social-institutional therapy and as many other activities as they can. I have never understood how they can be considered capable of making such judgments when they have had no formal education in fields of the complexity of the whole person, body and mind. Their attitude seems to be that the mind controls what goes on in the body, and they forget that the brain is a part of the body.

NEUROPSYCHOLOGIST and DOCTOR of PSYCHOLOGY

There are a few newer educational programs now which grant a Doctor of Philosophy in Neuropsychology, or a Doctor of Neuropsychology to candidates who have pursued studies toward a Ph.D. in Clinical Psychology but who spend at least one year of their education in programs which study the neurophysiology of the brain and central nervous system. Their research is limited to sensory and motor functions of the central nervous system and very rarely to the basic sciences of how the central nervous system functions. Most such Neuropsychologists are more interested in doing research than they are in clinical work with patients and often clinicians use them to establish a cause of a dysfunction by testing the patient to discover how much of the patient's malfunction may be "organic" as determined by psychological testing. They are not allowed the responsibility to interpret examinations done by Computerized Tomography (C T) and Magnetic Resonance Imaging (M R I), Positron Emission Tomography (P E T). Spectographic Proton Emission Computerized Tomography (S P E C T) as such newer tests require much more knowledge of neurology, radiology, and physics than that to which the psychologist is exposed. He does not study such basic sciences whereas the psychiatrist, neurologist and radiologist do in their medical and specialty training. Our ability to detect physical and chemical changes in brain functions is greatly enhanced by these new techniques. Such new techniques are not available everywhere in the United States, and some of them are used only for research, but it won't be many years before they will be readily available. The SPECT is a modified MRI and could be more readily available if the increased cost would be acceptable.

PHYSICIAN'S ASSISTANTS and ASSOCIATES

In recent years an intermediate level of professionals has been created called Physician's Assistants or Associates. Such professionals must be employed by a physician and are quite restricted in the functions they perform in accordance with the laws of the particular state in which they practice, and that varies from state to state. They usually study two years after having received a Bachelor's degree in programs which are similar to medical school, but are abbreviated to two years. I know of no circumstance in which they act independently to perform psychotherapy, or prescribe all the drugs which a physician may use. They may not do surgery, nor obstetrics, independently of a physician. It is very unlikely that you will be attended by a physician's assistant, but it might be wise to look at the certificates on the wall, which by law, are required to be displayed.

PASTORAL COUNSELING

Many ministers of almost any faith function as Pastoral Counselors. Probably the epitome of pastoral counseling is the confessional, where one goes to be forgiven of one's sins. Many Pastoral counselors do marital counseling and family counseling of a general nature. Many are members of various Marital Counseling or Family Counseling organizations along with Psychiatrists, Psychologists, and Social Workers. Some such organizations confer a "Certification" on their members. Virtually all pastoral counselors are members of the National Pastoral Counseling Association. The National Pastoral Counseling Association is not restricted to any particular religious denomination.

There may be other specialized pastoral counseling associations which are restricted to particular religious denominations but I feel certain that their pastoral counseling education is equal but frequently it is somewhat restricted to the particular religious denomination which the minister professes.

This does not make them significantly different in terms of the techniques which they use but it does make them somewhat different in terms of the interpretations which they will make to their clients, since the interpretations they make may reflect their particular bias as to their religious denomination and it's beliefs. A psychiatrist's interpretations also reflect that individual's personal beliefs and persuasions.

There are a few who have had Sexual Counseling training and do Sexual Therapy. Sometimes it is difficult to identify the type of counseling the Pastor does from the advance knowledge one might be able to obtain from customary sources. Most of the time the education the Pastor has received to qualify him for counseling has been in Pastoral Counseling internships of one or two years, as well as what he has learned from his professional organizations. Most Pastoral counselors are required to attend continuing education hours every year to maintain their skills in counseling in accordance with the latest Pastoral Counseling theories.

SOCIAL WORKERS

Social Workers are the most numerous of our professional ranks and are one of the most recent. Prior to about 1920 the profession did not exist. Dr. E. E. Southard of Massachusetts General Hospital sent out registered nurses to visit with patients and families in their homes to follow their progress. From that simple beginning Smith College in collaboration with Massachusetts General Hospital and Harvard Medical School undertook to organize a two year program for nurses in preparation for their tasks of observation. The basic curriculum devised in 1922 has not significantly changed, but an entirely new profession has evolved from it - now known as Social Workers, entirely separate from the medical profession and no longer requiring the social worker to be educated in nursing.

Those early social workers were not so professionally individualistic as the present ones. They were trying to do a job which needed to be done- save the physician's time in evaluation and in follow up in treatment. The great depression of the 1930's brought them into their own and they began to split off from the profession of medicine. Now, with two years of graduate work after a Bachelor's degree, they often feel that their contact with social studies prepares them to treat people psychologically on an individual or group basis; since emphasis has gradually changed from individual to group responsibility, social workers have come into their own. It is possible to obtain a Ph. D. in Social Work or sociology but the most commonly acceptable degree is a Master's which requires two years of graduate study in a school of social work after the Bachelor's degree. Most of the schools of social work in this country are dependent on departments of welfare for scholarships to keep their academic ranks filled. Yet, after graduation from a series of very general courses in behavior and sociology, many social workers feel they are qualified to be the equal of the physician in their capabilities to modify behavior of individuals in either individual or group therapy. They are required to complete "field work" which requires detailed individual supervision by Licensed Social Workers approved by the Faculty of a school of Social Work during the course of their academic experience. Many feel that they are no longer ancillary to the profession of medicine. Social workers are now certified or licensed in various states and undertake to modify behavioral or personality patterns of people. They have no education with the intricate complexities of the relationships between body and mind as they are not formally exposed to education about the body. Rather they are limited to a greater extent in their education than are psychologists. Yet, they frequently set themselves apart from medicine and often establish a private practice of counseling, as they have the benefit of legal sanction through certification or license.

To my knowledge neither psychologist nor social worker has rarely been called to legal test for professional ineptness, or malpractice in exercise of professional judgment. Yet, some set themselves equal to the physician in professional expertise of counseling and some courts recognize their testimony as valid as that of the psychiatrist. There have been a few court decisions challenging social work practice in specific situations. In the event that the pen is mightier than the sword perhaps words can do more damage than the knife.

NURSES

In recent years graduate registered nurses (Bachelor's Degree in Nursing) or registered nurses with an Associate Degree have begun to branch out on their own to set up clinics for individual and group psychotherapy and in some instances for some types of physical treatment. Usually such nurses have had some kind of specialized training or experience in group therapy or specialized clinics and feel that as a result of their personal maturity from their professional experience they are capable of conducting their own clinics for therapy - usually it is group therapy. I have no way of judging their competence to conduct therapy as most of that type of training in either self taught or is sanctioned by a particular group of cult like therapies. Formal nurse's training does not usually include instruction in psychotherapy although it does include some study of psychology and psychiatry, from a nursing viewpoint. Some independent practitioners have achieved legal authority in some states, to establish practice on their own without the usual requirement that they be in the employment of a physician as for many physical ailments. In a few states they are licensed to prescribe limited types of medications but not to do surgery.

Gradually over the years the philosophical attitudes about medical treatment have changed. Traditionally the physician is educated to treat the patient for the sake of the patient. A second goal is the treatment of the patient for the sake of society (as in many mental and correctional institutions or infectious diseases). A third alteration has now occurred politically as well as in the field of public health, ie: the treatment of society for the sake of the patient - as in evidence the political push currently in progress to create a National Health Insurance Plan. The fourth consideration is the alteration of society for the sake of society and that is what communism is all about.

Many comprehensive mental health centers as established under Federal Law now depend on social workers and psychologists to deliver "psychiatric" care. What few psychiatrists are available are often residents and frequently the only contact such residents have with patients is in signing prescriptions. Some psychologists try to direct the physician in the administration of drugs by preparing the prescription for the signature of the physician. Any physician who signs such a prescription without making his independent judgment about the patient is, in my opinion, guilty of poor judgment. Yet, such practices are followed on a daily basis. The advance preparation of prescriptions is a very common practice in tax funded mental health centers and in my opinion represents a gross degradation of the quality of care. In the end it is the physician who is held legally responsible for the prescription - be it of behavior, medication, physical therapy, milieu, individual psychotherapy or group psychotherapy.

COUNSELORS

There remains another large group of "psychotherapists" or "therapists" or "counselors". These are the people who achieve a Bachelor's Degree in some type of "counseling", most often the Departments of Education with a Bachelor's Degree in Education, major in Counseling. Some continue their education, often on a part time basis, and obtain a Master's Degree in counseling. A few continue to the Ph.D. level. The original intent of such programs was to prepare teachers for the role of counseling high school students in their high school curriculum. Then such people were added to the college or university levels to assist the students in selecting the proper courses for their major studies in college.

Now, they have branched out from such practical goal beginnings to feel that what they obtain at the Bachelor's or Master's level prepares them to do counseling with people who suffer from all kinds of adjustment problems, and perhaps with problems of living in general. Many such people populate the professional ranks of Community Clinics, and frequently are found in private practice. They, too, have virtually no education in the integration and complexity of body and mind.

LICENSED PROFESSIONAL COUNSELORS

Some states have established licensing provisions for "Licensed Professional Counselors" which most frequently is a definitive degree in Professional Counseling at a Master's Degree level. The curriculum may require several thousand hours of personal supervision doing counseling with "clients". As with all such educational programs, even with Allopathic Medicine, the emphasis of the theory taught and practiced at any particular University is that reflected by the faculty of that particular institution and such theories are wildly divergent, varying from a quasipsychoanalytic system of Freud to Gestalt theory of Bertram Lewin and others. This degree is particularly attractive to many people because it usually renders the counseling practitioner legally independent of psychiatric supervision.

PSYCHOMETRISTS

This is a group of people who usually have a Bachelor's degree in Psychometry. Psychometry is the art of administering psychological tests. Most such people do not practice independently and are not thought to be competent to enter private practice and I know of no state in which they are licensed or certified to enter into private practice although I feel certain that in some areas of the United States that some of them may do counseling.

Most of them are employed in state social services or clinics which are operated with funding from the federal government or from the state departments of social work or social welfare or whatever it is called.

The limitations which these people have in terms of the psychological tests which they are capable of administering are relatively great.

Most of the time the course work which they have completed to get their Bachelor's degree is taught only by other counselors and very rarely either taught by psychologists who have extensive training in psychometrics or by psychiatrists.

Under these circumstances, particularly the so called projective psychological tests which are very difficult to interpret, may be very poorly administered and very poorly interpreted even though the people who do it really feel and believe that they are doing a service to the clinic and to the clients who are referred to them.

One of the largest areas of difficulty is in the area of trying to establish some kind of organic brain syndrome or organic central nervous system malfunctioning as interpreted by such psychological tests.

The so called tests for organicity are very complex and require a great deal of skill in interpretation and frequently people with this kind of educational background have not been exposed to those kinds of learning experiences which would make them skillful at interpreting organicity from the psychological testing.

As I indicated above, most of these people are employed in the public mental health clinics and many of them are employed by the school systems to administer tests of the scholastic aptitude or tests which are presumed to measure a student's scholastic achievement. In many circumstances the tests to determine scholastic achievements are administered by the school teachers themselves and not by people formally trained to do Psychometry. Often such psychometrists perform complex tests of intelligence and the results of those tests follow that student throughout the course of his education through high school.

However, all those people who do administer such tests are very sincere individuals and they feel that they are really making a contribution to the world at large, particularly the children whom they are serving.

CERTIFIED ALCOHOL AND DRUG ABUSE COUNSELORS

There are a number of programs which certify Counselors in alcohol and drug abuse. Most of the persons who seek such certification are themselves reformed alcohol and drug abusers. The programs are certified by organizations organized to provide that certification. Such organizations establish their own standards for educational experience for the certification, and a specified period of time being supervised by a certified drug and alcohol abuse counselor. Usually only the experience and supervision under a certified counselor is acceptable toward the award. Should the candidate have experience under another person with different education, even psychiatrists, the award will probably not be granted. Yet, there are many individuals who avidly seek that certified designation as that means that they may be paid through government programs which fund treatment of alcoholics and drug abusers. Many of such certified counselors have only a high school degree or diploma as formal, acceptable, education.

CHAPTER 3

Each of the professionals whom I have described in the previous chapter is required to present his credentials and have them available on public display wherever it is they practice their arts.

In this instance, for example, we start with physicians. Physicians are always required to display their license to practice medicine in the state in which they are practicing and they usually have on display all the other credentials they have earned in the process of getting their education and those awarded during the course of their professional activities and practice. Having gone through medical school they should have a diploma from a medical school. They should have a certificate of their internship or residency. They should have a certificate of the specialty board in which they are certified to practice that particular specialty, in this case psychiatry, for which they are purporting to sell their time.

One of the difficulties is, that just because those credentials are hanging on the wall and you can look at them and examine them doesn't mean, of course, that those institutions exist, nor does it mean that those institutions are themselves fully accredited to bestow those credentials on the physician. However, there are other ways of finding out whether the physician is honest in displaying his credentials.

What you can do, is recognize the names of the various institutions which are represented by the credentials themselves.

Also, on that wall, or maybe more than one wall, there should be various and sundry papers and certificates which indicate that the physician has participated in his professional associations by his membership. In most professional organizations the highest membership category to which he can be a member is called a "Fellow" regardless whether the physician is man or woman.

There may be other kinds of certificates on the wall from the activities he may have had in the community. If he was on a board of directors somewhere, or if he had been a director of some organization, or director of a clinic, or something of that kind it is usually customary to present him with a certificate as to the service he had rendered while he was serving in the capacity of director or medical director or whatever it was.

Usually however, if he is an active member of a teaching faculty, he probably will not have a certificate indicating that he holds a special academic title in a teaching institution. You can take that for granted if he tells you.

But don't take too much for granted because if you really want to pursue verifying that he is what his certificates display he is, go to a library and look up the institution, university or other organizations which are represented by those certificates on the wall and which state he was in to receive that certificate.

Most reference sections in a library of a medium sized town will have some references which will include biographical data. Some libraries may not, but most may, regarding physicians.

Or if you want to go further you can call the county medical society or the state licensing board and inquire whether or not he holds a license. If the county medical society gives you reassurance that he is a member, that he does have a license, that he practices a particular specialty and what his educational background is, you can rest assured that at least the certificates he displays are accurate as to what they represent and therefor he probably is a responsible physician.

This gives you some assurance that he has had the training which he purports to have had and to give you more certainty that he has been exposed to the kind of education which you are seeking to take care of you. Nothing can tell you how skilled a physician or psychiatrist he is. There is no data bank for that kind of information. There is no way to find that information out. Should you ask for or obtain patient references there is always the chance that the particular patient you talk with may have a serious prejudice one way or another. He may have been a good or bad physician for the other person and just the opposite for you. You can only find out how he is with you by talking with him yourself.

This is true whether the physician is an osteopathic, naturopathic, allopathic or eclectic physician or whatever it is. Usually the name of the institution will reflect the particular type of medical system to which he has been exposed in his medical education.

It is wise to look at the certificates to see if you can find one which tells you that he has had a residency and where that residency is located.

In relation to the other professionals whom I discussed in the foregoing chapter, each of those professionals should have a license if your state licenses them or a certificate indicating that they are registered in that particular profession which they represent.

They should have diplomas on the wall indicating that they have had education in that branch of learning and you have to make an assumption that the education has been competent to give them the training that they might need to serve you.

I know that this is true of social workers as well as psychologists.

In the case of a marriage counselor, he will probably have on his wall a certificate stating that he belongs to the National Association of Marriage Counselors or some other organization similar to that to indicate at least that he has been accepted in those professional organizations as being competent to perform those functions which he is purporting to be able to perform.

However, no such certificate stating that an individual of any profession who belongs to a particular organization gives that individual legal standing in the state in which he is practicing. Only a license or a certificate to practice issued by the appropriate state board authorizes that individual to practice.

States have their own system of licensing or certifying individuals to practice a particular profession and under all circumstances if a certificate, certification, or license is required in that state for that profession then be certain that there is a form on the wall which indicates that the individual is either licensed or certified for that particular profession, as the case may be.

In the case of a licensed psychologist there should be a numbered certificate on the wall indicating that he is licensed to practice psychology in that state and depending on the level of education he has received and what the state law requires in that state, he should either have a Masters degree in psychology or Ph.D., or a D.Psy. degree in psychology or one of the subspecialties of psychology.

It is not always necessary for him to have a Ph.D. in clinical psychology in order to have a license to practice psychology. He may have a Ph.D. degree in some other branch of psychology, such as research psychology, psychometry, consulting psychology, educational psychology or some specific branch of psychology in which he has received his Ph.D. degree. Some people who have licenses to practice psychology have degrees in education and that would be a D.Ed. or a Ph.D. of education, so that this would give you some assurance that this individual has had a quality plan of education which leads to that degree and that he has been honored by having been presented a document which he should have on the wall.

Be wary of those individuals who have a document which appears to be a photocopy of the original. He should have the original hanging on the wall and not a photocopy. The same thing is true of all licenses for all professions. They should be the original. He may have licenses on the wall for other states as well other than the one in which you are seeking his help. In the event that he has more than one office at different locations, he might have a photocopy on the wall.

In the case of social workers, they have a very strong organization, The Association of Certified Social Workers, (A.C.S.W.). Sometimes social workers have a degree in sociology rather than social work.

In some states there may be sociologists who have achieved licensure by the state boards of psychology to be able to practice psychology.

These certificates will give you some assurance that this individual in whom you are placing your trust has gone through the educational steps required to obtain the diploma or achieve membership in those organizations.

The fact that all those diplomas, "sheepskins", are on the wall doesn't give you any indication of how competent that individual is to practice what he is licensed to do. You very rarely will find a certificate indicating the type of theory under which he practices other than that represented by the organizations to which he belongs.

Other prestigious organizations, such as the National Association for the Advancement of Science, take in any professional individual from engineering, biology, psychology, medicine, archeology and many other sciences in the various divisions of the organization which is of itself a branch of the major organization. Certificates are silent testimonials to that professional's interests and activities after having received his formal education.

Also there are many national or state directories which include all of the individuals who are members of those organizations and frequently those directories contain biographical data regarding this individual's education and training.

In order to be listed in those directories, the individual is investigated by the editors at the time he is accepted as a member, so that the data in those directories can be considered reliable.

Many of the organizations are very general in their nature, such as the American Psychiatric Association, American Psychological Association, National Association of Social Workers, National Association of Marriage Counselors, National Association of Pastoral Counselors, etc. and that covers a broad field of the practice of "psychiatry".

The psychological association is similar. The American Psychological Association covers a very broad range of the various sub-specialties in psychology and different subspecialties all belong to the American Psychological Association. I suspect that at the time you get into the office in order to seek help that you will be so distraught that you will hardly notice those certificates on the wall but if you can pull yourself together enough to look and cross-check I think it will be to your advantage.

There are numerous unscrupulous people in the world, some of them pose as professionals in order to make a living and such people in all fields of professional endeavor and are what are commonly referred to as quacks. You don't have any way of demonstrating their misrepresentation unless you yourself follow through and check on them. There, also, are many fraudulent "educational" institutions who "award" almost any kind of a degree for a fixed sum of money with no class time required. They are "Mail Order" degree mills.

Frequently, the professional organizations may or may not be aware that someone in their community is practicing who is not entitled to practice, are hamstrung by the fact that the laws are very general and the licensing boards may not be able to rid the society of those misfits.

Unfortunately, there is no guarantee that, even with all the certificates on the wall, the professional with whom you expect to work has derived sufficient education on a long term basis or has maintained his educational status by continuing his own education after he received that degree.

In very few professions are there stipulations that in order to continue to serve in that profession that person must take competency tests at periodic intervals.

There are several specialty boards in medicine which require recertification periodically, anywhere from three to seven or more years. There are some specialty boards in medicine which do not require recertification but do recommend it.

I am not aware that there is any recertification process of any kind in psychology and I do not believe that there is a recertification process for competency for social work.

Generally speaking anyone who has been in their respective fields for a period of ten years, if they have been active in it, have accumulated a great deal of additional education after they received their degree and they have generally emotionally matured in the process.

Nonetheless, the particular brand of psychiatry, psychology or social work which they practice may not be suitable for what you need even though they may be completely competent in the type of practice which they profess to do best.

What you need is specific to you and what they have to offer, even though they are competent in their field, may not be what you need so that you should make your own judgment about whether or not you should continue to see that individual. Such examination by you may take you two or three interviews or possibly more before you can make a competent decision about whether or not you want to stay with that individual for further care.

You have to remember that only physicians are licensed to write a prescription for you. There are some states in which nurses are licensed to do independent practice and are authorized to prescribe some types of medication without the supervision of a physician. I would be quite suspicious of any non-physician who offers to send you to a family practitioner to get your medication or recommends medication for you when that individual has had no experience, education or background in what the medications do.

It is easy to get a very superficial education by reading literature, but taking the responsibility for writing those prescriptions gives the physician a much more sound experience in knowing what the medications are which he prescribes and if he does not know about them when you ask, you should leave him and go somewhere else.

With all these suggestions I've made regarding his credentialing it still is up to you to make your own decision about whether that individual and you get along well together in what you are trying to accomplish and whether or not you are getting what you are seeking.

Remember, you have only your disturbed personality to work with in order to make your personality less disturbed and that is what psychotherapy is all about. Psychotherapy these days most often includes an appropriate prescription as well as just going in and talking. There have been court decisions rendered that a physician who does not use medications in treatment of mental maladjustment is not practicing adequately. In the past month I have seen a report from Florida in which a judge permitted a psychologist to be sued for malpractice and ruled that a psychologist is not a mental health professional. (May 1995)

I feel that prescriptions in and of themselves should be directed to meet your needs and you should not take more medications than you need, in number or strength.

One of the problems that you have to be concerned about is what you think your needs are. What your needs are may really be quite different from what you think they are. Ultimately, which medications and how much medication you take is your responsibility. Your physician only recommends which medications you should take, and how much, how often. Such decisions are very difficult for you to make but make them you must. If you feel that the prescribed medicine is not what you want or need, don't have the prescription filled or don't take it.

Nobody knows themselves well enough to be able to tell a professional exactly what it is they need. You can not be sufficiently accurate to know what you need or how to get it. You have an opinion about yourself and what you need but in the event that the professional does not treat you in a manner which you think you need doesn't mean that that professional is incompetent.

Don't forget that that professional has seen a lot of people and those credentials on the wall mean that he has had some experience and if he does not have experience, even that to which he was exposed in his formal education, then you shouldn't be there in the first place.

In getting their education, generally speaking, they should have had the opportunity to make some self appraisal and hopefully to have found something sound in themselves with which to work with other people.

CHAPTER 4

Now that you have decided to go to a therapist (if you did decide and didn't just run to the nearest "therapist", "counselor" or the most publicized one) and you have had a thorough physical examination including various chemistries run on your blood to find out if you have any physical diseases which might be corrected, you will be expecting the psychiatrist to respond to your needs as you present them while you are in his office. You will expect him to listen to you and hear you in the manner which you want him to cure your ills. Or you will want him to make some single dramatic statement which will clear away all your problems.

He isn't endowed with enough Divine Power to accomplish that, although that is the end to which he will be applying himself as best he can. To you it may seem that he should have all the answers to your emotional questions at the time of your appearance. He doesn't know what those questions are except as you present them to him through your talking and emotional expression. In order for him to get a clue to your problems, you must be willing to convey your thoughts and your emotions as well as the content of what you are saying. How you are saying what you are saying is the product of all of your life's experiences until the time you go into the office. You have no way of knowing just what experiences in your life are those to which you are adjusting by the manner in which you speak. Nor can you remember all those events, people and the attitudes of the people to whom you have been exposed and to which you are reacting by the way in which you talk and what you say, feel and think. Not all, but many of those earlier experiences and people in your life are influencing you right now. The way you are managing those previous experiences as well as your present life is you. As I mentioned above, getting into that office may seem like the end of the world to you, as to you it probably means that you have lost your mind or you would not be in his office in the first place. More people fear the title "Psychiatrist" because they believe that if you go to a psychiatrist that you have to be crazy. So you talk all around what you are trying to say, and also try to prevent yourself from showing any feeling at the same time. Yet, the talk and feelings are the only data from which the psychiatrist can make guesses as to what your problem might be. What you think it is and what he sees in it may be quite different. What you believe you are saying and what you are saying may be different because the last thing we want to hear from ourselves are those events and feelings from which we are hiding and at the same time are trying to express. The entire process of "therapy" revolves around assisting you in being more honest with yourself in the expression of feelings and thoughts, without compromising your moral values in the process either to hurt, or make love to the therapist. (Kaiser) Wishes to hurt or love are a part of the treatment but the expression of the passion must be within the limits of the treatment situation. Problems begin when either you or the therapist carries out those feelings and at that point the therapy is damaged or even lost. If the relationship between you and the therapist becomes personal then the therapy has gone astray and cannot be effective.

When you try not to express the feelings and at the same time express the thoughts, you block the progress of the therapy. Or you might be too emotional and present all the feelings without having any idea where they came from- and have a difficult time accepting the fact that the psychiatrist doesn't know where they came from either. At the same time, in that first interview will be the nucleus of all your problems in a very disguised form. The therapist will apply his own thoughts and feeling into trying to understand what you are expressing in thought and feeling in terms of the particular theory in which he believes. The therapist has no way of knowing what you are trying to say except by guessing what it might mean, according to the theory he thinks he is using.

He doesn't expect anything of you except the production of thoughts and feelings. He doesn't expect you to know what you are talking about. If you knew what was bothering you and could make the changes necessary to adapt you wouldn't be in the office in the first place and wouldn't need help. The therapist can not read your mind, and you are reluctant to let your feelings out, whether they be anger, affection or fear. The most likely feelings you will be expressing are anxiety or depression. It is most unlikely that you will come into the office blasting the therapist with your anger because you would expect him to retaliate if you did, which is probably what most people would do. So you try to hide the anger but feel freer to tell him that you are no good and hope he will try to boost your appraisal of yourself by telling you that you are worth something. At this point what you feel you want is sympathy and you may get angry if you feel he isn't supplying the sympathy you think you want. You may feel that he isn't any good as a therapist when you are so unsatisfied with what you feel you are not getting.

Most of the time what you feel is tension - anxiety and the feeling you are falling apart or will blow up, or will cry yourself to death.

The therapist usually doesn't know what to say and anything he says will only interrupt your train of thought and feelings. It isn't necessary to "dig" into your past for memories which you cannot conjure up. Digging up memories is impossible. Memories come to you as you talk about the present and they present themselves in very unexpected and tangential ways when you, or he, are talking about something else. If the therapist is comfortable with you he may offer you some piece of his life's experiences at times when you least expect it and may not want them to intrude. Or you may not understand how what he says has any bearing on what you are talking about. He rarely says anything without a motive to stimulate you to continue or to explore your talk in a slightly different line. He knows that he cannot coerce you into remembering. At best, all he can do is lead you into seeing some aspect of what you are saying which may be a little different from what you are seeing in it, or feeling, at the time you are saying it. He can't make you recognize, or feel it. His job is telling you what you have been trying for years not to hear about yourself.

Remember, he has no expectations and no more ways of conveying information to you than you to him. He is only trying to get you to expand your horizon of communications that you may see yourself in a different perspective without embarrassment. When you can do that and take an appropriate action to alter the situation in which you find yourself in the real world, the therapy has come to an end.

The entire process is only to let you learn how to expand yourself and be wary of those people in the outside world of whom it is realistic to be wary and to trust those who are trustworthy, and to learn to know one kind from another depending on how they react to you on a moment's notice. His sole goal is to help you be more realistic about yourself, what you are feeling and to assist you in the expression of that feeling, within the limits of propriety. He is not there to personally supply your emotional needs. Particularly if you feel the need to be loved - or to fight.

The therapist should be comfortable with his biological assignment, which includes his sex and that may tell you more about the therapist than the therapist knows about himself. Therapist's have to be comfortable, real people or they are not good therapists. If they are not comfortable they will try to coerce you into thinking that in their office there is only a one way street; that you are an unfortunate, confused person, and they are special. They are not special. They are just people like you who, hopefully, have undergone some kind of a self examination similar to that to which you are trying to expose yourself by being in their office. It makes no difference whether the therapist had personal treatment himself or whether his emotional stability was achieved by himself - only that he achieved it.

If it gets to the point in the office where the therapist makes some kind of affectionate or angry response you should be able to recognize whether you have stimulated that response or not. You will probably be unable to make an adequate observation that you want him to love you as though loving you would make up for the hurt and frustration you feel or to be angry with you and treat you as though you were an errant child. There are also times when you may want to feel comforted but whether that therapist can comfort you with words or not, depending or your state of desperation, is problematical. What he does do to comfort you may seem to be too little or too much. Too much in that you may begin to suspect that he has ulterior motives in what he does. What he does may seem inappropriate, ineffectual, or not enough and you are likely to feel angry. When you are in the passion of anger, crying, feeling lonely, misused and abused, or unloved, you may be unable to focus your attention to judge whether the therapist is taking advantage of you in trying to comfort you. In this state of desperation you can be vulnerable to his attentions, and that is when his moral values come into play. Yet, if you do not lose some control over your emotions, it is not likely that you will achieve the resolution of your problems in the long term. Be wary of a therapist who tries to get you to blame your feelings on someone else- parents, friends or relatives. You are responsible for your own feelings and the therapist is responsible for his own feelings.

None of these powerful expressions is likely to occur during the first interview. It takes some time to develop the depth of trust needed to let loose the degree of emotion necessary to change. Remember, the therapist cannot change you- he can only provide a climate of trust and hope for you to recognize how you have been managing yourself now and in the past to arrive at your present state of need. The only expectations he has are that you will be able to let some of the barriers down that you had been developing during the life you had before you came in for help. If none of the barriers come down - and it isn't necessary to shout, cry, or touch him to let the barriers down, he will try to loosen the bonds which hold your emotions in by making some remark to show you that he can withstand the emotional expression, or behavior.

The methods of adjustment you had developed in living had a positive survival value at sometime in the past. What brings you into the office for help is the fact that those methods of adjustment no longer have a positive survival value and are now preventing you from making an adequate adjustment. You had not developed sufficient flexibility in adjustment to change with the tides of living as they came up. So it isn't necessary to "dig" into the past to find out how you came to be the way you are, but only to understand and accept the way you are now that you may be able to make the change necessary to be more comfortable now. It is impossible for you to "dig" out those memories, events and reactions just because you want to here and now. You can only get them out when they are connected to something in the present which you can recognize, and you can't determine in advance what that will be. Neither can the therapist.

Some people, and some therapists believe that it is not possible to understand how you came to be the way you are without delving into your childhood to resurrect the childish and infantile experiences and memories on which you are basing your adjustment patterns and methods of expression of your feelings. I believe that it is entirely possible for you to make very satisfactory future adjustments and find much more facile methods of expressing yourself and getting satisfaction without ever having to dig up any of those childhood or infantile memories. There is always a possibility, also, that the memories that you "dig up" are those which you conjure up in order to produce something which you think the therapist wants to hear and if that happens of course, it is impossible for him at that point in time to tell what is a fact and what is a fantasy that you produced in those feelings in order to please him.

You are not in there to please him. You're in there to rearrange your relationships with people in general and he is a pilot study for you and you have to expect him to have one foot on the ground even if the other one is on a banana peel or a void.

In the event that the psychiatrist offers to provide you with a prescription to help ease your tensions he is doing that to help you to a quicker relief if he can. Prescriptions do not change your fundamental attitude but they do help correct whatever physiological imbalances in your nervous system contribute to or are caused by your state of emotions. It is not possible to have any feeling or emotions without having physiological processes going on in you. They are one and the same.

We (psychiatrists) don't really know whether the changes in our nervous system are the cause of our emotional disturbances or are the result of them. The body, and mind, have not yet told us that through research so we try to make the best of the knowledge we have and apply as much of our knowledge as possible. The entire situation is a chicken and egg problem. Psychiatrists don't know if one or the other - nerves or mind - is first or if saying nerves or mind is just a different way of saying the same thing. Certainly our mind can only work through our nerves and other physiological processes but at levels in the brain of which we are not aware. Nonetheless, those more primitive levels of the brain control and modify great masses of behavior while our higher levels seem to fine tune our social and behavioral functions as well as our receptive and motoric ones. At the same time our distance receptors connect to the "midbrain" through our cranial nerves and from that level the impulses are sent to our higher levels. The first contact we have with the outside world through our distance receptors (eyes, ears, nose) is at the more primitive level in our brain. At the same time the sensory reception we receive is mediated and modified by all our hormones and other chemical processes which keep us alive.

You must remember in the development of your whole body, and particularly of your nervous system, it is not completed at the time you are born. It gradually becomes more completed with the laying down of what is thought to be insulating material called myelin. There is some evidence to the effect now that some of the neurons in the cortex do not have their myelin laid down until you may be five or six years old. Under these circumstances of course you're still very much of a child and it's impossible for anyone, any person at that age to interact as an adult would. Although it is also true that whatever has gone on before all of the myelin is laid down and is in some manner recorded somewhere in the more primitive brain structure and you are probably making use of it in that portion of your thinking and your behavior of which you are not aware. (Cooper, Bloom and Roth)

So, trust your "hunches" when you first meet a newcomer, including a new therapist or psychiatrist. In order to trust your hunches you have to have some of your suspicious antennae on alert while at the same time trying to convey what is bothering you. The therapist should expect you to be suspicious, and not too trusting during that first interview, or perhaps for several interviews.

So far as the therapist is concerned, he wants to be paid for his services, but he has no wish to make you over into his own image if he is a good therapist. If he isn't a good therapist you should get out of there in a hurry. If you don't feel comfortable with him, leave. If you allow yourself to get so buried in your own feelings that you leave your judgment out then you will have to trust him, at least for that interview. Some therapists are very unscrupulous and the only reason they want you in the office in the first place is to collect your money and they will do what they can in order to keep you coming back to collect your money.

If you don't have your antenna out and question whatever is going on in there, in terms of how the therapist is relating to you, then you are going to be very vulnerable to his manipulating you in his own way for the sole purpose of keeping you coming back so that he earns his own living. If he makes his living by manipulating you to believe everything he tells you about how badly you were mistreated now or as a child, be suspicious. He is trying to get you to blame your adjustment on someone else, now or earlier in your life.

As you go along in the process of therapy you will gradually get to feel more comfortable with him and feel that there is a "give and take" in the therapy sessions including chastising him if he misses the point you are trying to make, and takes it in entirely different way than you intend. You will also accept his fumbling attempts to tell you what he sees is going on in you without your taking it as a criticism, but rather in the intention in which it is meant - a different way of looking at the same mental material. He is not trying to criticize you - he is trying to show you a different way of looking at yourself and your methods of expressing yourself. He doesn't advise you what to do. Any therapist who advises you what to do is imposing his own standards, or what he believes his standards are, on you and that he has no moral right to do. If you could have followed advice you probably would not have been in the office in the first place. Your neighbor or best friend has probably told you what to do or what he or she thinks you should do.

THERAPY IS NOT ADVICE. ADVICE IS NOT THERAPY. Remember, the therapist has no expectations- he is only there to tell you about yourself as he sees you and to help you be more honest with yourself in recognizing your feelings and in expressing them within the limits of social acceptance. He may try to urge you to make a greater effort in a direction of adjustment which you had not tried before, but whether you do or not is up to you. When you do try to react differently to some event or person you will be scared because other people's reaction to your new way will be unpredictable . You won't know what to expect and you will be anxious. You developed your present system of living to reduce that anxiety and at the same time to try to get some satisfaction for yourself in the process. What is unknown is usually frightening because we make it so. Don't forget that when you went into the office, the adjustment that you had made had survival value at the time you had to make the adjustment, which may have been anywhere from yesterday to the time when you were only a year or so old, or less, right after you were born. The reason you are in the office now is that the system which you developed to make those adjustments is no longer effective. It is time to leave it behind and find a new system of adjustment.

One of the paradoxes of such a book as this is that I am now advising you and it is entirely likely that you will not follow this advice either, because it is advice and does not permit a direct emotional interchange between you and I. It is difficult to express emotions by written words alone; the best writers can do is describe, and hope that our word pictures are accurate enough to stimulate a similar emotional, empathic response in the reader.

Therapeutic goals are often dictated by the conditions of various physical disease states which you bring to the therapy and which you may not want at all but which exist. You might only go to a therapist to assist you in accepting the limitations which your physical illnesses impose on you and that is a perfectly legitimate set of goals to seek. If you don't want to change your personality, don't try. The therapist should be able to accept the limitations you put on the therapy and should not set those total therapeutic goals for you - he has no professional or moral right to encourage you to get into therapy at a level which you do not want nor seek. From time to time it will be necessary for you to look back on the therapy to compare what you were like when you started and what adjustments you have made in the process of therapy. That is a legitimate examination for both you and the therapist. He may be doing the same thing with himself if he is honest with himself. You should always be in the drivers seat in the contacts between you- he has no right to impose his goals for you on you or to try. You are the boss.

The one thing he does expect is to be paid for his services. What medical insurance you have to help defray the expenses of the therapy is your insurance, not his. You are responsible for paying him, not the insurance company. If you are over sixty-five years old or are on Social Security Disability or Medicaid the Government may have already imposed the fee he may charge you, but if you wish to pay the bill yourself without involving the government that is no longer your privilege. If you expect the Government to contribute to the cost then both you and he are bound by their rules even if you dislike them. He may not like them either but he is, as a professional, as helpless as you to change the rules. Only congress can do that, or the regulators carrying out congressional directives to regulate, which has the force of law.

Just remember that if the therapist has only the expectation of being paid without the expectation of making an emotional interchange with you in order to help you change yourself then get out of his office because what he will do is try to get you to come back whether you need it or not and in order for him to be able to get his money. It doesn't make any difference who is paying for it under those circumstances. (Szasz)

It is also true however, that without some dependency on him, and without some trust in him that the effect which you want to occur cannot occur. Don't get to the point where you are so totally dependent on him that if something were to happen to him that you could not carry on your own life wherever it is at that point. What ever happens to the therapist, your life goes on.

Don't forget that the therapist himself also has some forces going on in him of which he is unaware. This condition exists in every therapist. No therapist is without nooks and crannies of his own personality which may need to be improved. When those nooks and crannies of the therapist's personality get in the way then the therapist may be doing things of which he is unaware which can foul up the therapy. What the therapist believes of himself may not always be exactly what is going on.

The only real expectation that the therapist should have of seeing you is that he expects to make a living out of it, but also if he is honest with himself he will do what he can to get you to a point where you're able to function much better than you were when you came in and to assist you in whatever way he can to arrive at that point so you can leave the therapy.

The therapist in a sense is like a good parent, or like a different parent, at least, than you ever had before and that is that the goal of every adequate parent is to get their children to a point where the children are able to function on their own and have some emotional and financial success in life with the satisfaction which goes along with it.

Fierman, Louis B., & Enlow, Allen; Eds.
<u>Effective Psychotherapy</u>
The Contributions of Helmut Kaiser
Free Press, Boston, 1965

Cooper, Jack R , Bloom, Floyd & Roth, Robert H
<u>The Biochemical Basis of Neuropharmacology</u>
Oxford Univ. Press, N.Y. 3rd Ed. 1978 6th Ed. 1991

Szasz, Thomas S.
<u>The Ethics of Psychoanalysis</u>
Basic Books, N.Y. 1965

CHAPTER 5

One of the major difficulties in adjustments which we make can be the inability, the lack of concentration, or the delay of thinking until after we act.

If our particular adjustment pattern is such that we act first and think afterward then we are in very serious trouble. I characterize such people as action oriented rather than thought oriented.

If we are to make use of our brain in it's maximum capacity it is necessary for us to put our brain in gear before we put our muscles in action.

Unfortunately, sometimes we are incapable of thinking before we act because our hormones, physiological systems or nutritional imbalances predominate. Then it may be that our brain cannot be put into gear first because of the lack of capacity we have to control what goes on. Then we are more likely to act than we are to think.

Thinking doesn't get people into social difficulty, acting does.

The problem with acting is that it is the actions that count in terms of the society and what lands us in court. It also gets us into using various psychedelic drugs, including alcohol and tobacco, in any form. Until now it has not been illegal to use tobacco but that seems to be changing and tobacco is banned in many circumstances. Nonetheless, acting first and then thinking is what laws are all about and gets us into trouble.

There are no laws to prevent us from thinking anything we want to think. Laws are in place to maintain some semblance of balance between people in terms of their actions toward one another. This also means an action which can be interpreted to be a contract, or the interpretation of an agreement we made with somebody, violates what other people would understand that agreement to mean.

Virtually all social institutions contain those people who act first and think afterwards.

Barroom fights, for example, where under the influence of whatever people buy in the bars that they feel they enjoy, may lead to an erosion of their capacity to control their action processes adequately enough and they end up in some kind of battle.

In family fights where murder, harm, mayhem, broken furniture, may occur are all the result of more capacity to act than the capacity to think and when it gets to the point where the action comes first and the thoughts afterwards then the damage that is done is always more severe than it is if the thought comes first, when there is some control over our actions.

The circumstances in which psychedelic, "mind expanding" drugs are used we have loosened control over ourselves by the use of a substance which is foreign to our natural state. Either that or our natural state has been damaged through our genes, infection, tumor, trauma and poor nutrition that it is necessary for us to correct what ever imbalances occur before we can do any correct thinking. Unfortunately, we are usually the last to know that our thinking is out of balance and then we act first and maybe think so seldom that we are not as adept at thinking as would be good for us.

Thinking can be crudely compared to making use of the resident software, or firmware in a computer.(ROM) Whatever we have placed in our memory banks might be available to us to review and consider what the results of potential actions might be if we take them, assuming that we are able to gain orderly access to them. In the event that we have used various mind damaging drugs we may not be able to do very much thinking in an orderly fashion. It is hard to recognize the typical identifiable parts of an egg once it has been scrambled. That's what happens when we use drugs- scramble the delicate physiological processes which go on in the brain constantly, and rearrange them, or destroy them in a totally unforeseeable pattern- or with no pattern at all. We also create a similar kind of effect when we use prescribed drugs but with the prescribed drugs it is hoped that the effect created will be of some benefit in constructively changing our physiology to remove some obnoxious feeling or chemistry which has already gone awry. Such as relieving pain.

Pain is a normal signal to the body that something is wrong and when it gets to be too persistent or severe we want to be rid of it so we take a "pain killer". Thinking we want to get rid of the pain is the first step. Then we take the action to take the pain killer which may or may not have been prescribed by a physician. Many are sold "over the counter" having been released for uncontrolled sale by the drug regulating agency of the particular country where we are. The drug we select may or may not have the "action" which we seek depending on what kind it is, what it does in the body, how much we take and how often we take it. It may have an entirely different effect that we expect, and may have more than one effect. The so called side effects may be more uncomfortable than the original pain of which we are trying to rid ourselves.

Should the drug we take loosen our ability to control our actions of thinking first and we impulsively strike out at someone because of a brief irritation the result may be more devastating than withstanding the minor anxiety or discomfort of the original irritation. The "side" effect of provoking the other person may be fatal, depending on how that person reacts. We may be less injured than being dead but we may be more uncomfortable than we were to begin with. (Not only does getting the black eye hurt but the black eye hurts much longer perhaps than the original irritation would have lasted).There is also the possibility that the person who we irritated by our impulsive act may reinforce his natural strength with the use of a lever, a club, a knife or a gun. In which case we could be a much worse loser. There are also times when a substance foreign to our body may be used against us by oral ingestion or injection. (an animal bite which poisons us is the use a "needle" which that animal had developed through evolution and usually injects a "foreign" substance- a poison). Such exchanges of activity constitute an action. All of us perform many kinds of non traumatic actions every day- without actions we cannot survive as we have no power to move or change anything by thought alone. Yet, injudicious use of action is equally as dangerous as no action at all, depending on the circumstances.

Our bodies may perform automatic actions for us to rid us of noxious substances for self protections. Nausea and vomiting from stomach irritants are such examples. Our reflexes, such as brushing off a fly may be automatic. Diarrhea is an automatic complex action of the body to eliminate foreign material in the intestines, such as bacteria, poisonous chemicals and toxins. Blinking is also one of such actions and is the fastest single action our body makes. If we don't blink at least once each fifteen minutes there is something wrong with our nervous system as even the minimum frequency of blinks is built into the protective mechanism to keep our eyes clean and moist for clear sight.

Since thought has been described as experimental action it sometimes helps to take such experimental action and think. When sitting around seemingly with not much going on, why not experiment with thoughts to ask ourselves what would we do if a given set of circumstances were to occur ? Suppose I ask myself what if I were to find myself driving in the rain and a car trying to pass me on a wet, slippery road starts to slide toward me as it draws even with me ? Or another car pops out on the left from a side road unexpectedly and the car on my left veers toward me trying to evade the car popping out toward him? What would I do ?

What if I find myself thinking that the world is not worth living in ? What am I going to do ?

In the example about the cars, I can imagine the various results if I were to take one action or another: veer to the right; go into the ditch on the right; slam on my brakes and possibly skid out of control on the slippery surface; shut my eyes, stiffen and let the crash happen with me helpless or any combination of these possible actions. What I imagine might happen if I take any of the experimental actions in my thoughts might well save my life - or make me more miserable.

If I simply close my eyes and stiffen to let the accident happen, I might likely be very seriously injured as I would be totally at the mercy of the actions of the other drivers. Should I panic and swerve to the right to prevent a crash, I might lose control of my vehicle and fish tail into the other cars or go uncontrolled into the ditch and perhaps overturn my own vehicle.

If I take the third option and slam on my brakes, I might be hit from the rear if someone is following more closely and could not stop - or even if no one is following me, my brakes might lock and take me to the right or left with the possibility of an uncontrollable spin which could create a massive pile up with all the other cars.

Suppose I apply some braking power, enough to slow my vehicle to a stop but not lock the brakes, and at the same time veer slightly to the right to the side of the road, but stay on the pavement ? I could possibly avoid the crash for the car on my left, as hopefully, he would be traveling faster than I and would continue on in a line straighter than I and so could pass me without making contact - avoid being tail gated by the car on my tail should there be one, maintain control of my steering and perhaps end up in the ditch but with a more controlled stop, much less likely to turn my car over. It is possible that the other cars might have passed me by and created their own mess without having me involved.

Not all the possible effects can be speculated because what happens to me depends upon what action the other drivers take but having thought about it once with the possible combinations of actions the other drivers might take and the conceivable effects which could occur, I may have at least imagined the worst possible scenario about what might happen to me and perhaps have created an experimental "thought path" to action to save myself from more serious injury. A lot would depend on what the other drivers did and if I had taken the effort to extend my own fantasy to give myself the benefit of the multiple scenarios from which to select one on which to act in reality to act more quickly and more safely.

Just suppose I wondered about what I would do if I got so nervous that I couldn't sleep at night? That I would feel so jumpy or depressed that I thought about what I would do to get some relief? I could tell myself in my mind's eye that I would go to see somebody and if so who? A neighbor? My wife or husband? The woman, or man across the street with whom I occasionally have lunch? The guy, or girl, at the next desk? My minister? or my doctor? or look somebody up in the 'phone book? But if the last, Who in the 'phone book?.

By going through this mental exercise I may arrive at some more reasonable action before I decide that life is not worth living and take a handful of pills, try to hang myself from the ceiling light fixture or drive my car into a wall. However, in order to take some more reasonable action I have to have one part of my thinking apparatus experiment in day dreams to look at my potential more rationally before I take any action in reality. I have to allow myself the privilege of questioning that my emotional state might not always be as pleasant, or as bad as it seems now. I must allow myself to imagine what it would be like to be different.

If alcoholics were to take such experimental action to imagine the befuddled condition they create in themselves and the upset stomach, headaches, inability to walk a straight line, or so dizzy they can't stand up, they might just not take that first drink. The problem arises that they take the action of taking that first drink before they think about what it will do to them. Unless of course, they like what that first drink, and the subsequent ones, does to them.

Not all actions are impulsive. Writing this book is an action. Starting it required a lot of thought and effort but the end result is an action. Whether it is a constructive action remains to be determined. Not all actions are quick and over in a moment. Many are prolonged and sedentary not making use of huge muscle expenditure of effort.

Many actions are social in nature, not just individual and personal. The recent blockages of various abortion clinics required the mentally coordinated effort of many people but the end result put muscles of many people into action . Yet, the planning took some time by a few individuals who recruited others to the scheme as time went past. The final actions became rather violent and opposed the law. Not to be in agreement with a particular law is acceptable thinking but as soon as one takes direct action against those who are operating within the existing law, that action is not acceptable because of the direction it takes. If the strategy were to inform the legislators of your dissatisfaction with the existing law and its interpretation by the judiciary, the protesters might have taken their action in another direction. They could have organized an action to encourage other people who hold the same opinion as themselves to petition or address the legislators to change the existing law, which would have been just as major an action as their direct defiance. Just to think and plan an action is not enough. It is also necessary to think about the direction the action will take to accomplish one's goal, which requires more thinking.

Planned action has to be commensurate with the long term goals at which you are aiming so there may have to be planned stages of action as well as short term action goals.

As a result of any action, whether it is planned or impulsive, in all probability there will be reaction. You must also consider that you are responsible for what you do. If what you plan is never put into action there is no problem but as soon as the plan is activated there will be responsibility whether the action is planned or impulsive. It makes no difference whether the action is successful or not, once it has been taken it is already too late and no excuses will suffice to undo it. You are responsible if you participated. However, many people who take part in such mass protests seem to feel that they are not responsible for having participated because, after all, everybody else was in it too. As though "everybody else" were to blame for their individual participation. Which amounts to say " not me, it was mob rule" . You have the option not to be a member of the mob as well as participating. The fact that even one other person also was involved does not relieve you of your actions or your responsibility for and to yourself.

However, nothing is accomplished without action. Coming into an office to find out what has gone wrong with you is an action. The first step toward consulting some one, whether it be the neighbor, or a professional is an action to help yourself which leads to helping yourself. Such action is taking the responsibility to rearrange how you will manage your life from now on. The process is slow and in trying to rearrange yourself the goals you set for yourself are never so clear and the steps to reach those goals are never so precise and definitive that you can plan them precisely because you are not aware of what motivates you to act as you do. If you were aware of what drives you to continue to behave as you have you would not have gotten into this mess. You are showing responsibility for yourself and proceeding as well as you can at this moment to fulfill a goal to reach a new you.

CHAPTER 6

Reality is what the world is and not just what you or I would like it to be. It is not what I would like to be but what I am, with all my personal characteristics, including my limitations. It is not what you would like it to be in your idealizations, but what your characteristics are with your limitations.

Reality includes all the plants and animals of the earth, the seas, the heavens and galaxies. It particularly includes all of mankind wherever they may be, in which ever country they may live and whatever their culture, deities, or circumstances of their existence. It includes the feelings of each existing biological entity and for all we may know the feelings and the existence of all the nonbiologic objects whether we are aware of their identity or not.

Our, yours and mine, capacity for conceptualization of the various complexities of living is seriously limited. We don't know what we are, what we do, nor how to do what we might be able to do or might like to do. Our ability to do is limited. Our ability to think and conceptualize is limited; our ability to feel and empathize with our fellow creatures is limited. Yet, socially we are responsible for what we do and for ourselves. We are unable to totally care for any other living thing or object because of the complexity of nature itself. Yet, try as we may we rarely feel, in our ignorance, that we are responsible for ourselves even though we are.

In an attempt to bring order out of social chaos, governments, laws, and social institutions have been created, in order to regulate ourselves and others.

Somehow, individually, we always feel that we are different, more special, than any other person, living thing or inanimate object. To each of us we are. I am more special to me than anyone else. You are more special to you than anyone else. In spite of this self centeredness there are occasions when we may sacrifice ourselves to some imagined benefit of someone else. At the same time, such sacrifice is often the superficial concept. Beneath it we may feel that by sacrificing ourselves we gain some advantage in our after life - heaven or the "hereafter". Each and every culture has this concept and hope, although under different names.

Whenever we feel that we have lost control of ourselves, we feel we have lost control of the world since we are our world. Then if we become anxious, depressed, angry, insomniac, overeat, gain or lose weight, develop aches or pains, over sleep or begin to blame everyone or anyone else in the world for our troubles we do not feel that we are responsible for what we believe are our troubles. At this point we are in trouble, of our own making.

As children we may fear we will not survive if one of our parents dies. Yet, the separation and divorce of our parents may be more frightening than the death of one. Death is real. Divorce is contrived, a social event not a real one. As children, we have much less control of our world and that is extremely frightening. Hopefully, as we "grow up" we gain the feeling that we have more control over our world and can make whatever adjustments are necessary. Also, to be aware of the events around us that we may be better able to interpret what's happening in order to put it to our advantage. We do not want to be a victim of circumstances. We want to be in control.

It is when we feel that we are not in control that we seek out someone else to help us regain that feeling of wholeness. What we feel at the time is the fear, anxiety, or major physical illness which may put us to bed with what we believe is real physical illness. Such physical illnesses can be caused by our attempts to make adjustments in the world when we have lost control of ourselves and which dominates our feeling and thinking. We are not really aware of how we came to be that way, unless it is in direct response to a recent life's event. Even then we feel helpless to change the course of events and our feelings. At times, we grovel in our self pity feelings and don't want to try to change them.

It is at the times we feel helpless and buffeted by circumstances beyond our control that we are most likely to make mistakes in judgment about our future and make decisions which are not in our favor, nor to our advantage. Sometimes we make major decisions which we later regret but cannot undo.

There are other times when we become enthralled with the romanticism of what is happening and may make decisions which can be just as erroneous in our decision making as when we are going through a crisis. Consuming love can be as much of a crisis as consuming hate or depression, but we rarely feel that we are in a crisis when we are in love.

We often feel that we are in a crisis when we feel depressed, unwanted or hated. We can sometimes follow our uncharted path without really looking at the other realities in the world to try to assess where we are in reference to where we thought we would like to go and whether we have any chance of getting there on the path we had selected. To awaken to the awful reality that we have spent several months or years in futile expenditure of energy and effort trying to reach a goal which will avail us of nothing is a very frightening and fearful realization. Often it is very depressing. Under such circumstances thoughts of wishing to get it all over with may go through our heads. The difference is, not that we think such thoughts but whether or not we try to destroy ourselves. There are many times in our lives when we feel hopeless and helpless, and there are, or can be, many times in our lives when we are helpless and have to depend on someone else to do what they can to see to our needs. Our weakness is in not having the faith in ourselves to see that it is never too late to change directions and strike out for a new goal in spite of the effort it may take.

To strike out toward a new goal means that we have to evaluate our situation as it is now and estimate our present methods of adjustment so we know where we are and what we are.

What we are is the system of adaptations we have utilized to arrive at our present situation. Many of those behavioral devices we have adopted without knowing that is what we have done. We unconsciously copied the behavior and attitude of some one during our growing years. Not necessarily copied someone who we admired, but perhaps at times copied someone who we did not like and began to behave in a manner which was not to our benefit. Sometimes we copied bits and pieces of many other people's personalities with whom we have been in contact. We had copied those traits to meld them into what we are. Everybody copies bits and pieces of other significant people from our growing up.

What's more, our personality never seems to stop evolving regardless how we live, or how old we get. When we stop learning and evolving we die. It is a constant, continuous life long process.

Reality is all the fragments, the bits and pieces of what I am trying to depict now. The conglomeration of all that has happened to us and all that which we have contrived to have happen to us to bring us to the state we are in at any particular moment in time. We are not aware of what all those bits and pieces are to have formed us into what we are.

It is not necessary to trace down all the fragments of our mannerisms, opinions, tone of voice and attitudes about politics, religion, way of life, expectations and the myriad of nuances of the personalities of other people to those friends or relatives from whom we copied or to identify them. That process is extremely long and wearisome. It takes a particularly persistent person to do that. In the process the "patient" may misidentify the therapist as those important people either one by one or at times fragments of different people at the same time. The therapist may also misidentify the patient as a different person in his or her life's span and that makes the therapeutic situation much more difficult. The "patient" expects the "therapist" to be perfect, and therapists are only people. All of these varied misidentifications and illusionary experiences are reality at the time they are happening and they happen to all of us from time to time and for the most part we are unaware that we are living them at the time they are happening.

It is desirable to identify the basic feelings which are generated in the course of the treatment and to keep them in context. It usually happens that the feelings come out as feelings, not just as words. There is no therapy unless the feelings do come out as feelings.

Therapy does not occur as the result of a discussion of the feelings. Which means that unless you get angry with the therapist, feel that you can't live without the therapist, will die if the therapist goes on a holiday, would like to kill the therapist for disappointing you in what life has provided, there is no effective treatment.

The counterpart of the angry feelings are the affectionate ones. It may be that you may feel that you cannot live without the therapist, and are "in love" with him.

Or that you could no longer exist if he were to die, and had become dependent on him for your survival. Any or all of these feelings may or can exist during the source of the treatment.

All such feelings exist in your mind and to which the therapist has not contributed other than by being there. Of course, that is assuming that the therapist has been "neutral" and has neither stimulated the feelings of affection, nor has become assertive or provoked angry feelings in you. When the therapist has been seductive or provocative toward you then you are only acting appropriately in reality to the stimulus when you become affectionate or angry. Therapy is thereby delayed in so far as investigating the basis for the expression of feelings in you. You are not able to separate reality from the internal emotional experience at the time it is happening. It is reality.

It is assumed, by both therapist and you, when you seek treatment that the therapist is "normal" and better adjusted than you are, which may or may not be true. Yet, at the time you seek therapy you are so desperate as not to be able to make an accurate assessment of reality and to make the appropriate adjustments to the situation in which you find yourself. So, for you, reality is so distorted in its assessment that you are not able to proceed in life with a sufficient degree of satisfaction without conflict with those people close to you or in society as a whole. When getting into treatment therefor, the therapist represents a microcosm of society so far as you are concerned.

All of which may be true. The therapist is a microcosm, a staunch, undemanding, accepting, protective piller against which to lean. Thus, at the time of coming into therapy you have relinquished your self assessment and judgment of reality and have sought the protection of the therapist.

All of the above considerations assume that there is no known physical disorder in you which is affecting your capacity to make judgments, or adjustments, and you are not being effected by the various organ systems of the body to stimulate or create a lack of judgment and the various symptoms which you bring to the therapist.

Physical problems often modify our emotional expressions. We don't feel that it is physical. We don't have a physical pain. Various viral infections over a period of time can cause us to react differently than we usually do. We just "don't feel right" get grouchy, depressed, irritable or intolerant of those around us. The result is that we become over emotional and overly sensitive emotionally but don't feel sick. To those around us we seem to change emotionally and they have a much more difficult time adjusting to our unusual reaction patterns.

The natural history of many viral infections includes a depression two to four weeks after we feel that we have gotten over the virus. If we jump into a long term psychotherapeutic relationship with a non-medical therapist during that time and undertake some suggested long term psychotherapy we can be making a big, unnecessary, expensive mistake. "Counselors" who are not physicians have no education to undertake to make an adequate assessment of what is happening to you under such circumstances. Nor do they have the education and knowledge to know how to investigate the possible causes of physical diseases. If your emotional reaction pattern is the result of any physical disease then that reaction pattern at that time might be better be left untreated as most of such reaction patterns are self limited and no treatment is either necessary or needed. Treatment of the physical disease would ease the reaction pattern, in which case no psychotherapy is indicated.

Similar causes of emotional problems are often associated with some kinds of heart diseases. Patients may present themselves with feelings of depression, insomnia, irritability or many other vague symptoms which on the surface seem to be emotional. Frequently in children who are having a hard time adjusting in school and who keep the classroom torn up with their antics, and the teacher at her wits end with their constant activity, may have a form of social seizure pattern which can be easily treated with medication and which does not respond to counseling regardless of who is doing it, or for how long. Reality is that physical problems can, and do, present themselves as emotional disturbances. It takes an astute physician to know how to discover the possible causes and interrelationships between the body and mind. The kinds of disturbances we are talking about are not uncovered with psychological tests because psychological tests can only discover what illnesses are affecting the brain and central nervous system directly, and not those illnesses which affect the rest of the body as well as the central nervous system.

Hormonal imbalances can cause similarly disguised symptoms as can nutritional deficiencies of the major food types and even trace element abnormalities. There are many different kinds of physical diseases which affect the entire body and can create problems in adjustment when the person involved is not aware that their reaction patterns have changed, but they may be very difficult to live with.

Reality is that we are very complex biological systems, and we cannot be separated into "body and mind" as though we were composed of those two entities somehow welded together but still separate in functioning.

What we are is the final whole product of functioning which includes our personality.

What we do to ourselves in the course of living also can modify our reaction patterns without our knowing it until it may be too late. For example: the use of alcohol or of the "mind expanding" "cool" drugs can subtly destroy our ability to adjust. What such drugs do over a period of time is kill off our neurons or greatly reduce their effective function and leave us to survive with less than "a full deck". They can also alter our hormonal balances, various kinds of metabolism and functioning of any or all organ systems, including our reproductive system. Those drugs which are commonly being used at present are some of the worst offenders in damaging our brains, hormones and capacity for the production of normal children. Marijuana is the classic example.

Recently it has been proven statistically that men who use marijuana and get a girl pregnant who does not use marijuana create the same statistical chance of producing a faulty baby as does the mother who uses marijuana. If both use marijuana the chance of an improperly developed baby is considerably greater.

Most people who use marijuana never realize that the more they use it the less astute their mental functioning becomes. There is no way to determine how much is too much for any single user. For some people even one joint is enough to significantly destroy their effective functioning. For others it may take years of frequent use to have that happen, but the only way to find out is to use the stuff until your brain fails. At that time someone else will tell you that your brain has failed, because having failed, your brain can not tell you that it has failed and you won't be aware of that fact.

Your partners in use will not know either as their brains will have failed at the particular rate for them and they may not be able to recognize that theirs or yours has lost its efficiency. You won't be able to notice that your partner's brain has failed for the same reason. Your emotional patterns will have changed so quietly that the subtle differences from day to day and week to week will have gone unnoticed as you will have made those changes without being aware of it.

The most devastating loss is that of judgment. Such loss or diminution of judgment is so subtle that when it is compromised we do not know that it is compromised because we have only the damaged judgment with which to recognize that our judgment is damaged, so we rarely recognize that it is damaged. Frequently there may be verbal battles in which we deny that our marijuana damaged thinking processes are damaged, and then only after some kind of disaster do we awaken to the fact that we were weakened. Recently a locomotive engineer of a freight train ran a red light on a track and struck a parked passenger train killing 16 people and injuring many more. The fireman is reported to have told the investigating officers that he and the engineer had been smoking marijuana in the engine cab just prior to the accident and that both were watching the signals and the track. Yet, they could not put into use the deep knowledge of the meaning of the colored lights and struck the parked train.

There are so many possibilities in life of events and adventures over which we have no control to influence the remainder of living for us that we are fools indeed to invite destruction by the choices we make. There are also times when we may not fully understand the implications of what choices we do make, and that, too, can be unfortunate. Nobody is able to predict the future, which is why so many people hope that they go to heaven when they die and may spend a great deal of time trying to prepare themselves for that event, and if possible to avoid going to the other place.

Until now I have inferred that the reality which impinges upon us is that reality which has to do with medical illnesses. I am certain that from time to time many of you have thought about physical disability resulting from injury which would interrupt your life's pattern. Here I will present some of the possible calamities, both of a social and physical nature which could change your life.

Under the category of social events are marriage, disappointment in love, divorce, death of a loved one, loss of a loved one from any cause, moving from place to place in the need to seek work, losing a job, or perhaps if your life style included the moving then stopping moving and living in one place which might be just as anxiety producing as for those who had stayed in one place and then had to move. Loss of property from a natural disaster, loss of money from a bank failure or just not having enough money to pay the bills and buy groceries until the next pay check.

Social and traumatic events of our lives might also be classified analogously to the medical terminology for medical and surgical illnesses. In the rubric of medical terminology all diseases can be crudely classed as Tumor, Toxic, Trophic, or Traumatic. Trophic being the changes which come on with old age and perhaps as the result of injury. Toxic meaning the influence of any infection, chemical or even poor nutrition to name a few. Tumor being any swelling, cancer, or any other sudden or chronic change in the size of various parts of the body, even from injury.

Traumatic may mean emotional trauma, such as the death of a parent, divorce, or loss due to chronic injury of a relative or even of a close friend as well as an injury, or any of the other social traumas which I mentioned above. The exposure to natural disasters may well require a sudden and immediate adjustment just to hang onto your life. Things like tornadoes, floods, volcanic eruptions, earthquakes, fires, or storms at sea or in the air.

The fact is that throughout life it is necessary for us to constantly make adjustments and usually the more unexpected the event which happens the more confused we are at the time. Sometimes the sudden realization that a pattern of events had gone on for a long period of time so we "got into a rut" and hadn't really realized how we had been behaving and adjusting to whatever life style we had, is a great shocker in itself and takes some time for us to reassess ourselves and to identify what happened, as well as how we had reacted.

All and any of these circumstances might lead you to conclude that you needed some help to cope with the strength of the tensions you go through.

On the other side of the coin, some people are so frightened of living that they seek out any minor deviation from what they think is normal living, or ache or pain, or swelling and they exaggerate what the reality is to a point of demanding that some physician or therapist agree with them that they are pathological when in reality their reaction to the simple circumstance is over reaction to a small stimulus.

Such people usually react too quickly to look at what is happening and make a rational appraisal of the event or circumstances in order to decide what is the appropriate thing to do. Rather they respond with their emotions rather than their heads and may find themselves in worse trouble than they were at the start. Such people are also difficult to live with because they over react to the interplay between themselves and their living partners and eventually the living partners just want to be free of the wild fluctuations of emotional response, and they are literally driven away by being overwhelmed by feelings.

Psychoanalytic psychiatry, Freud's metapsychological and psychological formulations of structure, content and form of the mind as well as instinct (libido), aggression, ego, unconscious id and superego all may be expressed has having a substance, form and perception analogously with clouds in an otherwise cloudless sky.

Like clouds they seem to have substance and can be perceived and studied as to their various shapes, sizes, colors, configurations, perceived height from the viewer situation and speculation from that distance can be made as to their composition.

Like clouds they can be modified by the winds surrounding them and other natural forces of nature including the amount of moisture in the air and other elements of the air which may or may not be natural to the air. For example clouds may be formed of vaporized chemical substances which are not normally found in the air in the concentration which they might be in that particular location. Such metaphors do not study the clouds themselves as the clouds can be modified, dispersed or concentrated by the forces of nature impinging upon them. Psychoanalytic psychiatry has similar qualities. The consistency of mind, dreams, hopes, emotions, feelings and thoughts can be molded and changed by the winds of psychotherapy and I use the "winds of psychotherapy" intentionally. However, the nature of change is very indirect since the winds of psychotherapy must be integrated, received and subsequently modified. The underlying forces of neurophysiology which may be modified much more quickly and definitively by the more direct application of other simple or complex chemical substances such as medications.

Just as clouds can be dispersed or concentrated by more direct and guided applications of forces of nature other than the winds impinging on them. Various types of drugs can alter the forces of nature much more quickly and effectively than just the winds of psychotherapy alone.

However, one of the problems of the use of drugs in the reality of treatment is the fact that there are very few drugs which do only one thing and perform only one function in the body. At the time drugs are ingested or injected they affect other organ systems in the body as well as the mind.

Neurophysiologically, they have an affect on all other organ systems which are called "side effects". All drugs have "side effects".

Side effects sometimes are utilized to a more efficient extent to perform some other function on other organ systems after the drugs have been in use for awhile. What were originally viewed as being side effects then may become the primary reason for the administration of the medication. With this in mind reality becomes a loosely defined conceptualization. Loosely defined in so far as psychotherapy is concerned because the "winds of psychotherapy", namely, the movement of air, the movement of optical rays, even smell, all of the distance receptors which in impinging on their respective specific receptors within the central nervous system must make the same changes in the neurophysiology of the individual as drugs if a person's personality, their fears, their emotions, their conceptualizations are to be changed. The same "natural" physiological changes have to occur whether they are made to occur with the "winds of psychotherapy" or medications. Effectively, the reality of the situation is that it makes no difference how these changes are received by the individual's complex physiological mechanisms, the ultimate change has to come about on a neurophysiological level.

One of the other complexities in this analogy is that there are times when the distance sensory preceptors do not record what is happening accurately. For example, hallucinations might be considered to be an antidromic receptive process (it goes in the reverse direction from normal) which causes the hallucinations to be real to the individual having them. It is almost as though the neurophysiological processes which are stimulated produce the hallucination, voices, visions, tactile sensations or even misplacement of body limbs in proprioception.(That kind of nervous signal which tells your brain where your body parts are in relationship to each other and in space).

To make the situation even more complex, both audio and visual sensory processes are fooled. Delusions can occur in what is actually out there to be received and seen or heard, may not be the true cause of the sound or of the visual impression. We may often misinterpret the reality of what is out there either to see or to hear. The sound which is created may very well be not what it is but it may sound like something else. Or our minds may associate it with some other object or event and misidentify it even though we may hear it accurately. When it comes to visual misperceptions, which we could call illusions, the relationship between two objects which we are viewing may be seen in several ways. What we are actually seeing does not change but our mind interprets it in two or more different ways depending on what the circumstances are and what the stimulus is.

Thus, if we are going to impinge on the neurophysiological processes by use of the winds of psychotherapy it is necessary for us to understand how the individual who is receiving those impressions interprets them. There is a myth that psychotherapy can do no wrong. Psychotherapy can do a great deal of harm due to the fact that what is done and what is perceived may be different from what is the cause of the perception. Even reality is a relative thing. What is not relative is the effect that the distance receptors have on neurophysiology.

Neurophysiology, in order to be functional, has to be the same regardless of what is stimulating it, whether it is drugs, medicines or the perceptions of the distance receptors. Plato recognized the complexity of conceptualizations and how man views the world in his allegory of the cave in which Plato very clearly pointed out that it is as though man is standing at the mouth of the cave with the sun behind him and that what man sees in the cave are the shadows which are cast on to the back wall as a result of man standing in the mouth of the cave with the sun behind him. He, himself, can not look at the sun because of the strength of the stimulus so what man actually sees are the shadows of the real world and not the real world. That can be said of any of the distance receptors. What really doesn't change is what the reality of the real world is whether we know what that reality is or is not.

However, since our perceptions are based on neurophysiological responses it is not too significant what causes those changes. Unfortunately it takes a great deal longer with most people to cause those changes with the winds of psychotherapy than it does with medication even though the medications themselves are almost never as specific as we would like them to be.

Neither are the distance receptors as specific as we would like them to be and they too, as I indicated above, are subject to misinterpretation by the receiver and also they are subject to misinterpretation as to what is being transmitted by the individual who is transmitting.

We forget that psychotherapy does not mean only audio. It means visual and odorous as well and sometimes touch. Freud's attempt to reduce the sensory input by using the couch did not constitute a favor to his patients. One of the reasons he began using a couch with his patients was the fact that the patient was unable to see him.

Not all the alterations are necessarily for the better, whether the alterations come about by medications or by the psychotherapy. An inept psychotherapist can create as many mischiefs, difficulties and harm as a misapplied medication or medication which has undesirable side affects. Just because it is psychotherapy doesn't mean that it is all helpful; it can be extremely harmful if the psychotherapist doesn't have any idea or doesn't have enough knowledge or awareness to know what is happening with the patient as the psychotherapy proceeds.

Jowett, B.; M.A. The Dialogues of Plato 2 Vols.
©Oxford Univ Press Feb, 1920
4th Prntg. Random House, N.Y. 1937
Vol I. Rep. Bk. VII p 514 Pg 773

CHAPTER 7

Methods of therapy are as varied as the numbers of psychotherapists in practice. Many of the formal theories and treatment methods of managing the treatment are in print. Most psychotherapists believe they are following a particular theory when they practice. However, the facts are that what he does and how he does it is his own unique style. What the patients receive from him is his brand of therapy regardless of what the therapist thinks he is doing, or what theory he thinks he is applying. The only caveat which I believe exists is that therapy is NOT advice.

Advice is useless. It can be obtained from any neighbor, family member, friend or enemy. It is not worth the trouble at any price, particularly that of the "professional". If advice worked then no patient would appear at any office for treatment. By the time you have made the commitment to come, or have been sent by some social institution, you have already received appropriate advice from many different sources, and had heeded none or you would not be in the office. If you had heeded some of the advice you had received it might have led you to be worse off than you were before you received it. This is true because what you bring to therapy is a manner of adjustment to life in yourself which is not working and you already know it is not working. What you don't know is how to be different from what you are and to make the change to some other way of adjusting which will be to your advantage to make life easier, or at least a little less uncomfortable. You come because the tricks of adapting to whatever experiences you had in life are no longer effective and you now find yourself anxious, fearful, sleepless, depressed, aggressive, angry, in jail or in need of an alcohol and drug therapy program if you haven't already been to one. You may feel you are not acceptable as a sexual partner, receive no satisfaction from the patterns of adaptation you have been using, or haven't had an opportunity. So you feel like seeking a quick way to undue all your ineffective maneuvers to obtain the satisfaction you would like to have. You usually are unable to think clearly enough to examine what you are or who you are.

At the time you come you believe that what you want from the therapist is "understanding", acceptance and person to person relationship. Not sex, but affection and approval of you as a person. You also want to be relieved of your fears, anxiety, depression or what ever it is that you bring to treatment. If there were some way to "cut it out" analogously to what the surgeon does, in one interview or contact, you believe you would be superbly happy. That can't be done.

How the therapist accomplishes his miraculous cure is of no concern to you. You dump yourself on the therapist and want the magic to begin without any effort on your part.

"Effort" in psychotherapy means being willing to hear what you have been trying for years to shut out of your mind about yourself since those unwanted feelings are likely to come to the surface and be expressed more directly than your personality permits. The devious ways you use to simultaneously express your feelings and hide them is what makes up your personality, or leads to the symptoms which cause the trouble in adjustment. None of us likes to hear things about ourselves which we have been trying not to hear. It is emotionally painful. None of us likes to be emotionally pained, except in some unusual instances. If the therapist is a good one, he will focus on one of several techniques to promote the expression of feeling. Feeling is not something one talks about to express. Feeling is feeling, with force and passion. It is expressed but cannot be discussed with any therapeutic effectiveness. Discussion is intellectual evasion of therapy.

It is the expression of feeling to and with the person about whom some one generates feeling, or that person in the immediate presence who represents and is seen as a surrogate for some other important person in the past or present which is the basis of therapy. That important person does not have to be a parent, or relative. It may be the kid down the street where one grew up, or a fantasized relationship with a movie star from the distant past who one has never met. It may be someone in the present who does not share the intensity of feeling I have about him or her. Or, it may be that the feeling is shared but there are other interfering limits which prevent the full expression with each other. The substitution of the therapist for some other important person in the patient's life is what Freud called "transference". Transference comes about without the patient's knowing about it and when it occurs in reverse, i.e., when the therapist uses the patient in the same way, as a substitute for some one else in the therapist's life, it is called "counter transference". Transference and counter transference have nothing to do with the type of emotion which is expressed nor the form in which it is expressed, but only with the fact that it deviates from the reality of what goes on between the therapist and the patient.

I view hypnosis as a form of physical therapy. I view all and any form of "psychotherapy" as a form of physical therapy. Just as drugs are used to alter the performance of neurotransmitters for therapy, psychotherapy must do the same thing if therapy is to occur. We may abstract all we wish about our "minds" but the act of expression of thoughts or feelings is a process of the physiology of our central nervous system and its various methods of accomplishing what it does. That means we can only express our selves by the complex systems of interaction between the neurotransmitters, hormones and the local hormones and nerve complexes which are native to each organ.(Prostaglandins, nerve "rete", reflex arcs, local chemical secretions and reactions, etc). It makes virtually no difference what "psychological theory" is applied by the therapist the end result must be that physiology is changed and new, more functional and efficient physiological balances are created in the patient in order that the patient is "changed"

Psychotherapy is a physical form of therapy simply by influencing what goes into your various sensory systems, your distance receptors, especially vision, smell, hearing, in order for you to be able to change the interpretation of the input to be converted into neurotransmission in your mind and central nervous system. Processing of that sensory reception must be different from what it was before you began therapy, if therapy is successful. That being the case, in the long run I feel that physiological methods of altering such changes are involved in psychotherapy or in the use of drugs. At this state of our science we have little knowledge about how either system works. We can alter the workings of the mind faster with drugs than with psychotherapy, even though we don't know exactly how. (Barondes, Samuel H.)

Broadly, therapy can be medication, one to one contact with the therapist, group contacts or physical forms of therapy. Normally we all are members of multiple groups in the conduct of our life. What makes a group a group therapy group is meeting together for the primary purpose of mutually, consciously, changing our way of living emotionally. Therapy goes on in all the other types of groups as well but it is an indirect form of therapy, not the dominating force to bring the group together. You may be wondering why I put medication as a form of emotional therapy. Current knowledge, as incomplete as it is, does have some powerful medicinal tools which may alter the manner in which our biology functions and may be a short cut to changing the bases of the expression of our feelings, and the manner in which we think. Like all other tools it is not without some effects which may not be desirable, known as "side" effects as well as being ineffective in the hands of the amateur professional. It can also be dangerous in the hands of the amateur or professional if it leads to attempts at suicide, or an increase in overt aggressiveness toward other people. Furthermore, it may lead to a distrust toward other professionals if the relationship doesn't work out well and no further formal attempts at psychotherapy are attempted. I have not decided whether to call these people amateur professionals or professional amateurs.

So the family doctor may very well be prescribing emotional treatment when he hands you a prescription. If the family doctor is knowledgeable about the prescriptions he hands you, and is able to identify the major problems with which you are suffering, or the major symptoms, then everything may go well. Family doctors don't know everything either, so he may miss your particular situation and may possibly miss giving you the correct prescription for your condition. Not all medications for the same emotional condition will work with all people, which is a possible stumbling block. So he may have to try several different medications, any one of which may have worked with other people but not with you. In order to find the one to which you respond may take more time and experimentation than you are willing to tolerate. If it is possible, be a little patient when he is trying to meet your needs.

It is also true that to depend on prescriptions for the sole treatment of your emotional ills may be a trap in itself. It is necessary for you to reassess yourself to make changes although in many instances once the alteration has been initiated by a prescription and equanimity prevails that prolonged continuation of a medicine may not be necessary and it may be either reduced or eliminated with impunity. That depends on the kind and type of medicine it is and the difficulty, both emotionally and physically that you may have in reducing it or stopping it. Sometimes no other form of therapy will produce any positive results and it is necessary to continue medications for a long time, years. Nobody is able to predict the outcome when the medications are begun. In a significant proportion of instances no medication may be of help, but then, nobody can predict the outcome when individual or group psychotherapy is begun either. At times there may be no recourse except physical forms of therapy such as electroconvulsive therapy and that, too, is no guarantee.

I alluded to electroconvulsive therapy above. Since it was introduced about 1936 it has been used extensively, and continues to be used. Over the years it has been refined to such a point that little or no overt evidence of a "convulsion" occurs. It remains controversial but it works and sometimes produces a permanent relapse in symptoms, especially in depression. More often than not, it is used for depression after all other methods have been tried and failed. No method or medication is a sure fire treatment which will cure. At present E.C.T (Electro Convulsive Therapy) has as good a score in "cure" as any other method. It is painless and quick and should not be forgotten when all antidepressant medications have been tried and failed. Frequently it is suggested as a form of treatment for many other emotional illnesses and has proved very efficacious for many although it, too, is not a cure all. It is painless and quick. Electroconvulsive therapy has been shown to be a very safe and effective form of therapy where all other forms of therapy fail. It is not fool proof but neither is life fool proof.

Just as medication can possibly be interminable, at times individual or group therapy may come to be interminable also. Thus, regardless of the form of the therapy it is not without the potential for complications.

In the event that one to one psychotherapy leads to too close an attachment of you to the therapist, or the therapist to you, complications can arise. If you are unable to keep some emotional separation from the therapist then you may have a very difficult time bringing the therapy to an end. If the therapist is good he will make every effort to develop and maintain an emotional distance from you for your benefit. Frequently the kind of closeness in emotions involved in this situation are felt as feelings of "love". It is very rare that the therapy is difficult to bring to an end when the feelings develop around anger.

When anger prevails, that session or sessions, will probably be very stormy, and if it comes out too strongly the therapy may come to an end needlessly and emotionally harmful. You might not go back, or you might walk out, or say things which later you regret. Anger, frustration, anxiety, all can be a stepping stone to a better emotional adjustment. Not infrequently you may awaken several days or weeks later to the fact that you were out of line when you exploded at the therapist. Then is the time to renew your contacts with the same therapist and if the therapist is worth his salt he will accept your former explosion for what it is:a part of the therapy. However, many people become very ashamed of their behavior and feel unnecessary guilt about having treated the therapist in the manner they did and never make an effort to contact him again, thereby losing a significant portion of the possible positive effects of the explosive encounter. It is also possible that the hostility and anger generated is so deep that it is not possible to return to the same therapist which usually means that a very deep emotional attachment is beneath the anger.

Sometimes it is possible that your tension will become so high that you get up and leave the session in the middle, usually very angry. Most therapists will say something to indicate that they expect you to return at the next scheduled appointment about the time you are going out the door. If they don't say something, either call and check if you have an appointment, or assume that you do have and keep the appointment as if it had been regularly scheduled. In the event the therapist had not rescheduled you for an appointment you have realistic grounds to be angry which may complicate the therapy.

In some instances should you feel almost uncontrollably "in love" with the therapist and begin to feel that if you don't leave the situation you might end up in making love, leave that situation. You can always cool off and try to discuss your feelings at the next interview even if it takes you more time than the interval to the next scheduled interview. Call and tell the therapist or the receptionist that you need more time to collect yourself before you will be able to retain mastery over yourself emotionally.

Should you be a part of a group which is in therapy feel free to express yourself. If you do not actively participate you are defeating the very purpose for being there. Unfortunately the only assets and liabilities you have to work with are those with which you went into therapy. So in as much as you can not just drop your old attitudes and adjustment patterns just because you went for therapy they are all with which you have to work. So do the best you can.

Groups are organized by the therapist in accordance with the concepts of the therapist in reference to the theories in which the therapist believes. In this situation what the therapist does may not have any special reference to the psychological theory on which the therapist is basing his responses. The other members of the group are probably as ignorant as you as to the theory the therapist believes he is using. In these times the broad concepts of the various psychological theories may be common knowledge to some members of the group if not to you. Certainly with all the popular books that are available to present those concepts it is a pretty good bet that someone in the group thinks he knows what is going on or what is supposed to be going on. At the same time, how the therapist intervenes in the discussion will reflect what the therapist thinks he knows about the theory. The ideal situation is that the members of the group will interact with each other and the therapist can sit back and work his mind in an effort to interpolate how each member of the group is interacting with the other members.

When the therapist does intervene, it should be for the purpose of elucidating the process which is occurring and not with the idea that any individual member should have some element of his personal history brought into the open for the other members of the groups to share. Only you should have the option of bringing your own personal history into the group discussion. The other members of the group, as well as you, must have the opportunity to add their ideas about why you react the way you do to what has happened in the group at that time, or at some time in the recent past during some prior group session. You must feel open to make tentative suggestions about why others in the group reacted in the manner which they did. None of these observations of interplay between the members should be taken personally.

If one or another of the members of the group begin to feel that they are being picked on or attacked by the group or any of its members then the process of therapy breaks down and the feelings run too high to be of service. If someone gets mad or becomes overly attached to another member of the group the process fails. Invariably at different times and at different levels of reaction such outbursts may occur.

In all groups there is usually a requirement that the members of the group do not seek each other out for social contacts outside the group therapy sessions. Such "outside" relationships can carry over into the group sessions and present entirely new sets of circumstances to be dealt with during the therapy sessions. That may be difficult to do and may generate fragmentation of the group into factions and prevent constructive discussion. A show of feelings (crying or anger) in group often leads to sympathy from some members and denigration from other members with the result that the group becomes too intense and may break up, at least for that session. Ultimately it should be possible for all members of the group to accept such overt feelings without too much disturbance, but that is the goal of therapy and may take a long time in coming.

Other types of groups may be centered around activities wherein each member of the group participates in some communal effort toward a single goal. Each member of the group may "go off on his own" to do something different or cooperatively help in working toward the common goal. Most of the time in such a process the personal attributes of each member of the group will come to the fore and there may be interruptions to discuss why someone in the group did this or that. That, too, should be accepted in a spirit of helpfulness rather than a spirit of criticism. If any one in the group takes it as criticism then the cooperative effort of the group will suffer.

Some types of groups may be centered around each individual member of the group presenting a topic for discussion, or a short lecture on some topic of his particular interest followed by discussion. In these instances the prime purpose is to provide a stimulus for the members of the group to share their ideas and feelings about the topic chosen or presented. Feeling might begin to run high with the differences of opinion which invariably develop. When such heated discussions are taken personally and "sides" develop to strengthen one position or another then the group can fragment and become argumentative rather than cooperative.

There are many different kinds of groups for therapy. Just above I presented a discussion type. Some groups are organized around activities; some are organized around role playing; some are organized around reading and there are as many variations of the format as there are conceptions to create them. One type of group may not be suitable for you so look around you if you find yourself in a group which you feel does not fit you to find a group which does.

Group therapy, too, can become "addictive". When it does the patient or client goes from one group to another getting no help from any and always coming away dissatisfied. However, usually there is less anger felt about failing to achieve a cure in the group because there is no one person to "blame", only the non productive group. People don't blame a group of other people, just individuals, unless one hapless member of the group stands out in the mind of the disappointed member and that hapless individual gets the blame from all the others for the failure. A kind of "mob" blame. You will know about it if you happen to be the one all the other group members blame for the failure.

Electroconvulsive treatment, exercise, hormones and sometimes surgery can be as effective "psychotherapy" as any other methods, under some circumstances remember.

I saw a young woman who was unfortunate enough to have had lopsided breast development. One breast was an "A" cup and the other a "D". No amount of "psychotherapy", or psychotropic drugs would have altered her major embarrassment of that condition, as she had no control over her unbalanced state. A plastic surgeon altered her entire outlook on life, but she was about 30 years of age before she found the courage to bare her bust and share her embarrassment with a psychiatrist, or with a surgeon. The plastic surgeon performed more psychotherapy in an hour and a half or two hours than I could have done in ten years even though the lady never married.

To recapitulate some of what I've tried to say in this chapter, the individual therapist performs individually. Regardless of what the theory is on which he practices or of which he thinks he practices. What he actually does may be totally different from the theory he thinks he's following and that doesn't make it any less effective if he has a good self appraisal.

If you, under these circumstances, go away from such therapy believing that you have been exposed to a particular form or a particular theory and then you try to find out what all that theory entails, I feel that you are wasting your time.

It is true that the content of what the individual therapist tells you will be presented to you in the terminology of that particular theory as the therapist understands it.

Currently there is a fad, mostly among non-psychiatric therapists to blame sexual abuse in childhood or infancy as the cause of many of the maladjustments which occur. In my mind there is no doubt that some sexual abuse, or what is called sexual abuse, does occur on occasion in all cultures. On the other hand I feel that this fad of blaming sexual abuse leads the therapist into leading the patient into producing fantasies and other manufactured memories in the patient, because the patient wants to please the therapist. When this happens, of course, the patient is trying to please the therapist and tell the therapist what the patient feels the therapist wants to hear. When the therapist wants to hear about sexual abuse the patient produces a great number of false memories about sexual abuse. In extreme cases the patient then comes to believe these false memories, which have been created to please the therapist. Such false reality becomes a very major detriment in the conduct of the therapy, all of which the therapist has suggested rather than patient having actually experienced the sexual abuse in reality. When this happens, of course, the patient does not have any way of knowing and does not feel that they have deliberately misled themselves or the therapist into the false memories which they have produced. Those false memories then take on the quality of reality because the emotional driving force in the patient is to please the therapist. That doesn't always make it what the therapist believes it is.

Barondes, Samuel H.   Thinking About Prozac
        Science 1994; 263:1102-03:25 Feb. 1994

CHAPTER 8

The manner in which the therapist performs his art is entirely up to the therapist. There are as many techniques as there are therapists. One author who canvassed the various techniques arrived at thirty-six and then wrote a second book on the newer systems of psychotherapy. I am not trying to expand on his effort since many of them are variations of the same basic theories. What makes the techniques different is the manner in which the therapist applies them and what the therapist thinks they are. What is accomplished then is what the patient gets out of it and may be entirely different from what the therapist thinks he is doing, or is trying to do. The end result is that therapy is the peculiar brand of communication which that individual therapist uses. What the therapist is as a person is at least as important as what he thinks he is doing in therapy.

Broadly speaking there are five major forms of technique in individual therapy:

(1) Those which probe into the patient and make an effort to relate what and how the patient adjusts in the present to some significant person or incident in the past.

(2) Those techniques which focus only on the present and try to elicit more clarification of the feeling the patient may have toward significant people in the present.

(3) There are also those "behavioral" techniques which try to get the patient to behave, or react in a manner different from what they had done in the present, or if they can recollect the past, different from the manner in which they had reacted the first time and perhaps all the times in between when they had reacted that particular way under similar circumstances. Thus, the theory is that if they can change their behavior now, when and where

they began to react or behave in a particular way is not important. It makes a difference whether the therapy takes place in individual interviews or in groups. The desired goal is the same, but the intensity of the therapy is generally much greater in individual interviews than it is in the group setting primarily because there is a greater diffusion of feelings in the group to more people because it is a group. The one on one interview puts only two people in the arena of the office and that focuses feelings on fewer people.

(4) This does not take into consideration the fact that in the past thirty years a great many drugs have been developed and put into use which may facilitate the process of communication, by reducing anxiety or depression. In some instances the use of drugs may be all that is needed to allow you to arrive at your own conclusions and to modify your behavior and emotional expression to a point where prolonged interviewing therapy is not needed and may be detrimental. Only physicians have the legal authority to prescribe medication so if the therapist is a lay person (medically speaking) this avenue of therapy is not available unless you want to complicate your life more by seeking a non-psychiatrist physician to prescribe the medication. Many nonpsychiatric physicians who prescribe psychiatric medication do it without the detailed knowledge of the drugs they prescribe which also can become a problem.

Of course there is also a considerable number of psychiatrists who adhere to the old school of interviewing techniques and who refuse to prescribe medication. (Donovan & Roose)

(5) There are also some psychiatrists who adhere to another old school who perform various kinds of physical treatments, such as electroshock therapy, for many different forms of emotional disorders. There are

fewer of these adherents to EST (or ECT) than there have been in the past but there are some. Virtually no one does other forms of shock treatment anymore, nor are surgical procedures, such as prefrontal lobotomy, performed. It is possible to fall into traps at either end of the treatment scale and not receive a kind of therapy which might be the most appropriate for you. I remind you that only physicians may legally prescribe physical forms of treatment, although there are several groups who do use the body as a form of therapy, such as "Rolfing". In some cases Jacobson's "Relaxation Therapy", which also uses the body, is utilized. Most Rolfer's, hypnotists, relaxation therapists, acupuncturists, masseurs, encounter groups, etc are not physicians.

There are a great many people who come to therapy who are not able to make use of the "probing", talking, techniques in which the therapist tries to delve into the patient's past and makes interpretations of the content of the therapy which relate to the patient's relationship with some significant person from the present, childhood or infancy, or the feelings which were stimulated by a particular incident from infancy or childhood. Unless such associations come "spontaneously" from the patient the remarks the therapist makes may not only be ill advised, but may be harmful and lead the patient into the suggestion from the therapist which the therapist wants to hear. So the patient tries to please the therapist by producing such instances which may or may not have occurred in reality. When such productions from the patient occur, the patient believes them and they assume the same emotional charge whether they occurred in reality or not. The therapist may hear what he suggested he wants to hear but he has no way of knowing whether that particular production occurred in reality or whether it was concocted by the patient to please. The patient can't separate reality of past event from the present fantasy of what he thought occurred.

To complicate the situation even further, the patient may relate his fantasies which might or might not have occurred at the time of the said event, and may not be able to distinguish the fantasy from reality, now or then. To the patient the fantasies may be as real as any event which might have occurred. Such turns of events in treatment can be devastating for the patient since it helps them lose their grasp on reality and tends to reinforce the reality of the fantasy which they then take to be a real event rather than a fantasy. They may then proceed to produce more fantasies to which they attach the same emotional charge they attach to reality. The therapist is quite unable to distinguish the difference between the fantasies and the reality of the past, since all the information he has to use has to come from the patient. So a good therapist sits and waits until he has a sufficient amount of verbal evidence that the story or incident which was related was real or a fantasy. The sitting and waiting of the therapist often makes the patient nervous and he begins to feel that the therapist is not listening, doesn't care, is thinking about something else or isn't doing anything.

It makes no difference whether the patient is sitting in a chair facing the therapist (vis-a-vis), lying on a couch with the therapist at their head, or pacing up and around the room, the fantasies may come and go with the same complications.

Hypnosis falls into the class of psychotherapy. It is form of interviewing and in spite of what many people believe it, too, can produce as many false notions as any other form of psychotherapy. During the course of the state of hypnosis the patient may be partially aware of the need to please the therapist and produce fantasies which have no basis in reality. Memories may be falsified and the patient may believe those fantasized memories just as truly as he believes the true ones. The therapist has no method to separate the true from the false and is quite unable to distinguish between them.

One of the oldest forms of psychotherapy, acupuncture, began in the orient. It is a combination of invasive technique and suggestion because the needles do puncture the skin and are buried in the flesh. In the original technique they were "twirled", rolled between fingers to rotate and increase the stimulation. More recently small electrical stimuli are applied through very small wires to increase the stimulation. There is also a variation called acupressure in which finger pressure is applied to specified spots which is said to have the same effect as the puncture. For those who believe, it is a very effective method and sometimes it is said that Chinese physicians perform major surgery with no more anesthesia than acupuncture but recent visitors to Chinese hospitals have found that some form of western anesthesia is most often combined with the acupuncture.

There is an jocular form of therapy which sometimes angers those who believe they do "real" psychotherapy, called "Hug" therapy. This was created by a nurse who wrote several small books similar to children's books in that the "text" is cartoons with a bit of poetry to illustrate the circumstances under which a hug is beneficial to one's sense of well being. To qualify to be "Hug Therapist", one hugs. It seems silly, but it promotes good will and feelings of conviviality and is NOT sexual in the interpretations of the hugs. It works, unless of course, some rigid individual interprets all hugs to be sexual. In this time of sexual harassment it is quite possible that some individuals who are frightened of any body contact, even with clothes on, might misinterpret a hug in public to mean a sexual assault.

The use of the couch for psychotherapy, which Dr. Freud initiated and popularized because he was unable to tolerate having patients look at him all the time during the course of his routine therapeutic day. The couch was for Dr. Freud's emotional comfort.

He felt he was under too much of a spotlight as one of his reasons for placing a patient on the couch and allowing them to look at the ceiling. On the other, hand he positioned himself in such a way behind the couch that he was able to view their countenances so he could make interpretations, guesses, of what the patient's facial expression meant as it changed and the communications between Freud and the patient progressed. Thus, he created a visual one way street. He could see them but they couldn't see him. He felt that was a more equitable situation so far as he was concerned because by that means it was not necessary for him to be exposed to the patient's interpretations of his facial expression or movements.

We must remember that facial expression is not the only means by which a person may express their feelings. In his so called "body language" Dr. Wilhelm Reich initiated his Character Analysis. Dr. Reich interpreted the patient's position on the couch as well as their facial expressions to indicate to him that the patient was experiencing some emotion in relation to the body language of the patient at the time. The emotional expression was reflected in the patient's position on the couch, as well as the fine movements.

The end result is essentially the same whether the patient is on the couch or whether the patient is in a chair. Psychoanalysis is defined by the content of the therapist's interpretations of the verbal content the patient produces, not by the patient's position in relationship to the therapist.

It is an artificial social situation to have the patient's back to the therapist, in a straight or reclining chair.

In that instance the patient cannot relax as comfortably and thereby remove or reduce the effect of gravity on his body. Ordinarily one thinks of repose as lying down because in that situation the forces of gravity are distributed more evenly over the entire body and there is more of a chance that rest will occur which is one of the other considerations that Freud made when he first began making use of the couch.

It is also true that on the couch, the patient feels somewhat isolated from the therapist and many people feel that they don't have to face themselves when they bring forth whatever content they relate. It gives them an opportunity to more or less "hide from themselves" so that they don't have to feel quite so embarrassed about those circumstances of the content of which they may be talking at the time. So it helps the patient to feel a little more distance between him and therapist.

Sometimes physicians or other therapists will resort to a reclining chair as a substitute for the couch. This allows them to fool themselves into believing they are doing a form of psychoanalysis and at the same time not mimicking psychoanalysts so if anybody asks if they are analysts they can truthfully say they are not because they do not use a couch, as though the use of the couch were the distinguishing feature between one who is an analyst and a therapist who isn't.

Many people who aspire to be "psychotherapists" seem to believe that they can do no wrong, that psychotherapy cannot be harmful but they may do a great deal of emotional damage to the patient in their lack of appreciation for the emotional investment which the patient puts into the contacts. (I see that I have revealed my orientation by calling such people "patients" since most "psychotherapists" who are not physicians usually call them "clients".) Many psychotherapists may temporarily forget or not fully appreciate that it is the nature of the unconscious that we are not aware of it. When a discussion of the unconscious takes place there is no therapy and virtually no contact with the unconscious. The patient may feel that they are getting explanations of their behavior or of their thought processes, which in reality are not important. They may have gotten more out of their time and effort to have gone to a movie. The unconscious makes itself known in devious ways, but not by discussion of it.

When there is a meaningful expression of the unconscious it usually arrives unexpectedly, and with a significant amount of feeling. Perhaps enough feeling to disturb the conviviality and cohesiveness of that particular interview.

Feelings don't always express themselves as anger. Just as frequently they may express themselves as affection and dominate the atmosphere just as much as when they come out as anger. Feelings of affection can be more disruptive than feelings of hostility, and just as persistent and sometimes much more persistent. Feelings of affection can be more destructive in the long run than anger or hostility for the reason that feelings of affection may lead the therapist astray by promoting a personal relationship with the patient. Hostility may provoke a personal relationship with the patient but it usually is not a pleasant one so it has a tendency to bring itself to an end. Affection has a tendency to prolong itself between the partners because it is pleasant, and "makes one feel good". It can side track the purpose of the interviews into the prolongation and promotion of the personal contacts. When contacts get too personal, there is no therapy.

There is almost constant discussion, accusations, and "research" among "psychotherapists" as to whether or not sexual contacts between therapist and patient are appropriate. Sometimes "Sexual Contacts" are defined as hugs. Such research may get a lot of attention as journalists greatly enjoy promoting all kinds of adverse publicity toward "therapists". There is considerable doubt in my mind whether hugs constitute sexual contact. They may or may not be, depending on what they lead to afterward. Sometimes, more empathy can be expressed in a simple hug than all the words in our vocabulary and it is not desirable that they lead to more intimate contact. I have argued with some therapists whether or not the simple act of helping a woman on with her coat at the end of a session constitutes a sexual contact. I feel that simple courtesy, opening a door, shaking hands, assisting in putting on a coat is not a sexual assault nor suggestive of a more intimate contact. If a man were struggling with a big thick coat to find the arm hole, I would also assist him which would not mean that I am making a homosexual approach

. Each therapist develops what he thinks is the best method to approach and to manage the patient during each session and over all. Many therapists feel they have the right to direct the patient to think about some aspect of his life and assign topics to discuss in any one session or to direct the patient to complete a task during the intervals between sessions, as though the therapist had complete control of the patient's life between sessions as well as during the session. (Cognitive therapy)

Specific techniques and entire systems of treatment are designed around such approaches. What makes them work, when they do, is the belief the patient has in the therapist to be of help. Which technique is used is not really important. It may be more important to the therapist than to the patient. If a therapist has no faith in what technique he is using it won't be of help, so the therapist may delude himself into thinking that what he is doing is for the good of the patient, and believe that he, the therapist, has the only significant answer to solving problems with psychotherapy, and the resolution of the patient's problems. Most often the effect of the therapy cannot be adequately measured until some months or years after the patient leaves the office and has gone about his business of living on his own.

If the therapy really works, the patient will not remember the details of what happened but will be reconstituted in a slightly different emotional and behavior pattern which serves him well in living, but he may not remember how he got to be that way and will, more often than not, forget the therapist's name. Any therapist who has left the patient with a desire for further contact, or who has received several referrals from a former patient has not done his job. He has programmed the patient to make more money for himself by leaving the patient with residuals of unresolved feelings. Unless the patient had broken off the contacts, in which case the rebound might not be so positive unless in the breaking off the patient is ready to continue his life in his new configuration.

So, technique resolves itself and is defined by the personality of the therapist and not by the abstract theories of psychiatry which the therapist believes he is applying.

Some limitations of the techniques and application of the therapist to the patient's problems are indigenous to the reason or feeling which brought the patient to the therapist in the beginning. For example, if the patient goes to see a religious counselor because of confusion about his religious beliefs then the therapy would be expected to be limited to clarifying the religious confusion. Should the counselor begin to delve into the personality of the patient with the idea that the patient needs more detailed and deeper change in his personality which may have caused the confusion of the religious beliefs, then the therapist is probably delving into depths for which he may not be prepared. Under such circumstances he may cause more damage than help. The same is true of marriage counseling.

It is true that the partners in a marriage bring their own unique personalities with them into the marriage. In the event the marriage falters, then those difficulties may be derivities from the personalities which existed prior to the marriage. I feel that an attempt to investigate the personalities which existed prior to a marriage is hardly within the province of the marriage counselor for at that time the therapy has taken a new twist and has begun to lean toward individual psychotherapy of either one or both partners.

There are some techniques which assign "role playing" in the individual contacts, in which the therapist tries to put the patient in some one else's shoe's and asks the patient to respond as the patient feels the other person would under a hypothetical set of circumstances. Such techniques may be effective if the therapist takes into account that the patient, nor no one else, can leave their own personality behind in assuming the artificial role of someone else. Such play acting can only be colored by the patient's personality even though the patient may be trying his best to either incorporate his personality into, or separate it from, the role.

Entwined with all the talking is the possibility that a medication may assist in the loosening of tension that the patient might make more progress than without it. In the event that two people may be seen at the same time in interviews it may be helpful if both of them use some medication. There is no guarantee that the use of medication will help, nor is there a guarantee that not using it will help. There is also no guarantee that the particular technique which the therapist uses will help because in the long run the relationship which develops between the various partners will determine more how the treatment succeeds than any other factor.

Psychotherapy is only an impingement on the neurological mechanisms of the central nervous system through the distance receptors. A hug is closer and more primitive as it involves touch and may carry a lot more meaning than the stimuli through the distance receptors. A slap will also carry a lot of message.

Reich, Wilhelm   <u>Character Analysis</u>
Orgone Press, N.Y. 3rd Ed. 1949

Harper, Robert A.   <u>Psychoanalysis and Psychotherapy 36 Systems</u> (paper)
Prentice-Hall, Englewood Cliffs, N.Y. 1959

<u>The Newer Psychotherapies</u>
Prentice Hall, N.Y. 1975

Donovan, Stephen J., & Roose, Steven P.
<u>Medication Use through Psychoanalysis</u>
J. Clin. Psychiatry 56: 177: 5 May 1995

Keating, Kathleen
<u>The Hug Therapy Book</u>
Comp. Care Pubs, Minneapolis, 1983

CHAPTER 9

In each session you will wonder what to talk about. That will be especially true the first few times you go, which is a completely normal reaction.

After all, a psychotherapeutic session is an artificial situation in which you consult someone about your own life. One of the unrealistic expectations you will have is that you will expect to get some advice.

Under some circumstances, if your tensions are so high that you simply can't contain yourself, then you will begin spilling out your life's story without any prompting and when that happens of course you are already in the middle of your treatment, at least you've begun it.

However, the sessions are usually not as frequent as they used to be. In times past people often went to see their psychotherapist every day for four or five days every week. Now a frequency of once a week is considered pretty frequent.

The rules are very simple. Unless the therapist makes a suggestion that you talk about some particular topic you're free to talk about anything you like and whatever "comes to your mind".

All of us have a lot of ideas racing through our heads all the time and ordinarily we automatically select those which we will talk about and those which we wont talk about.

The goal in therapy is to get you to talk about all those little things that go through your mind that you reject as not being pertinent, not being appropriate, too volatile, and too emotional to talk about. Basically the quickest way to get to what's going on inside of you is for you to say whatever you can grasp of all those concepts and ideas that are going through your head so quickly and spit them out to the best of your ability.

If you feel that the speed or the feeling that you're showing is inappropriate and you don't let them out you impede your own progress.

In my opinion, there are certain rules which nobody should violate. Of course as a therapist, I don't like to get hit and I do not make an effort to try to seduce any patient of mine, male or female, into any kind of a sexual relationship. I think that of any such overt behavior on your part toward either striking a therapist or cursing him, cursing him is acceptable, striking him is not; trying to get him or her to make love to you is not acceptable and any therapist who gives in to those wishes, even though it may be very strong in you to be loved, is out of line. Then I think it's time for you to get up and leave. Unfortunately, at that time you are probably responding with your feelings and not with your thinking processes. If you become enamored of him and the therapist does not let you know that taking action to make love from such feelings is inappropriate then the therapist is either taking advantage of you or you of the therapist.

Another trap that comes about in therapy is just talking about medication. In this day and age any psychiatrist who does nothing but talk with you and does not offer to give you some kind of a prescription to help get you calmed down, less depressed, less angry, to get to sleep, or to help whatever the major problems are as you express them when you go in, is not performing his function appropriately in your treatment. If, because he had given you a prescription, you go to the sessions and talk about nothing but the adjustment of the medication dose, or the effects of it, you are diverting your time to topics other than therapeutic ones. You are using the medication as a shield between you and the therapist and are not using your appointment time well.

Most of what we know about the physiological functioning of the human brain is an extrapolation from animal brains but none the less, the total body of knowledge that's available to us now has been increasing by leaps and bounds. About ninety-five percent of what we know about how the central nervous system has been learned since about 1970 and under these circumstances the medications which are available are far more effective, even though there are a lot of scares about their being addictive and having severe unwanted "side effects". Most of them are not addictive on a short term basis.

You will find that some kinds of medications will make the interviews go much better and your life outside that office will be lived in a more satisfying and less tension producing style. The medications in and of themselves are not magic. They won't do the whole job without your sitting down and going over your own lifestyle and as Socrates said "The life which is not examined is not worth the living" so the fundamental goal in the long run is for you to examine your own life and that's where the therapist comes in.

I feel that it is not the therapist's job to give you advice. It's not the therapist's job to tell you what he thinks you ought to do. It's up to you to find out for yourself what it is you are doing that you are not being satisfied, how you are managing yourself that you're not satisfied and how you show to the world the manifestations of that dissatisfaction. When you learn these things about yourself then, you are the only one who has the capacity, and the option, to make what changes you desire to make within yourself. You can turn out to be more like the kind of a person which you would like to be. Unless one part of you can sit back and examine what you are saying, at the same time you allow yourself to say it, you're going to have a more difficult time.

The old psychoanalytic system of theorizing about all your adjustment system originating in your background from infancy may or may not be true. We don't know, as such theorizing is an abstraction of a system of thinking about how people get to function the way they do, which doesn't mean that you have to go back to remember all of those old memories, feelings, affects and ponder them, obsess about them, worry about them in order to change yourself.

On the other hand some of the newer theories about behaviorism indicate that what you do now influences what you remember from the past and probably influences the interpretation of your memories from the past. What the therapist focuses on of the content the therapist believes will influence you in the content which you talk about in the office. There's no way to avoid the therapist's interpretations but you don't have to agree with them.

Don't forget that the therapist is also a person. The therapist also believes that he or she is a professional and being a professional, many feel that they have a right to direct the therapy. If that professional feels that he has the right to direct the therapy, the kinds of questions he will ask, the suggestions he will make, the interpretations he will make, will all have a distinct bearing on what you talk about during your sessions.

One of the big traps when you go to see a psychiatrist is the fact that the psychiatrist will, in all probability, make some suggestions about taking medication. If the psychiatrist and you fall into the trap of talking only about the medication dosage, the nature and severity of the side effects what effects and what the problems are that you're having with your medicines and nothing else comes out, then you will be as much at a dead end as though you were trying to do formal psychoanalysis at one day a week in delving into your memory bank and trying to produce all those memories which may or may not have happened in order to relate to your infancy.

Either extreme, it seems to me, is cause for concern because the focus on one or the other of those extremes shuts out all the other possibilities of what might be going through your head and when that happens you are automatically limiting your own exposure to yourself, what you're thinking and what you're feeling.

Content also implies that therapy is an intellectual exercise. Therapy is not an intellectual exercise; it's an emotional experience. There's no way that you can avoid developing some kinds of feelings either toward the therapist or the therapist in his own way toward you at the same time.

If you hold back those feelings and try not to express them you will be impeding treatment. They are a part of the content of the psychotherapeutic experience and without those feelings the likelihood of there being any meaningful change in you is very small.

Of the complaint you bring, whether it be anxiety, depression, insomnia, whatever, are symptoms which represent an attempt on your part to manage yourself through your life and at the same time suppress some of the undesirable feelings which you have, at least those feelings which you feel are undesirable. You are simultaneously trying to express yourself. That being the case it's necessary for you to mobilize those feelings as well as the thoughts. Freud recognized this dual role of symptoms. There are very complex terms for it but the expressions of those feelings is absolutely necessary.

What you have to take into consideration is, that you are expressing them whether you realize it or not. What you are in therapy for is to find a more satisfactory way of expressing them both to yourself and to the world around you.

As you find more satisfaction in being able to express yourself you will find that you will be more direct. You will be open. You will also be more selective of those people with whom you do share your feelings and share your thoughts.

The pilot person with whom to study yourself and with whom to make your changes is the psychotherapist. That is what you're there for. You, of course, are dependent on the psychotherapist to do what he or she can do to accept you as you are and to help you make the changes which you want to make in yourself. If you have no desire to make any changes in yourself then there's no reason for you to be in the office in the first place.

I feel that it is a gross error for a psychotherapist to try to inculcate into the patients who come to see him what the psychotherapist feels their life should be. It is not the psychotherapist's business to determine what your life should be. Psychotherapists, in their concepts, may try to guide you in a particular type of adjustment and the interpretations they will make to you will be in the light of what the psychotherapist feels is the best thing for you to do or the best adjustment you might make. Should the therapist initiate these topics he is discussing your adjustment with you and thereby delaying the inevitable presentation of you to you. The therapist may be making it more difficult for you to take the initiative about that topic.

It is for you to determine what is the best way for you to be. It is for you to determine what is the best thing for you to do. Of what you talk about in there, you should make the selection. You should follow your own trails in your own mind.

I do caution that there are going to be many times when you will feel lost and you will feel that there are no trails to follow. In that case you have to be honest with yourself that you're having difficulty in accepting the fact that whatever is troubling you is deeply rooted in you, which it probably is, but you are afraid to confront your own freedom of expression in order to get to those feelings. They must be extremely strong or you would not be so fearful of them.

The psychotherapeutic experience is not an intellectual exercise. It will help you none whatever for somebody to give you advice. What will help you will be the interpretations of your actions which the therapist makes. The terms he uses in the interpretation of the expression of your feelings, the explanations of how the therapist feels that you came to be the way you are for that particular episode. It will not be of any help at all to you if in the content of the therapy there is a discussion of your feelings. In order for those feelings to be real and manifest it's necessary for them to be expressed. That means the feeling has to be real. It has to be felt by you and the therapist should be sufficiently emotionally stable and distant enough to accept the expression of those feelings for what they are. Your system of making what adjustments in the world which you have made and which you are trying to change you have developed over a long period of time. It's not something which just came to you overnight.

It's the fact that those systems of expression of feeling have lost their effectiveness is what brings you in for "treatment" in the first place. In the event that you fall into the habit of trying to please the therapist by telling him what it is that you think he wants to hear and try to imitate the feelings as though they're real but something that you don't actually feel to show him that you are in his corner won't work. You can't make up feelings and have them come out real and expect to change yourself. You've got to use the therapist as a real person. When those feelings do come out will be most helpful. When the feelings are real you will have impulses to either leave, get angry, make love, or you may want the therapist to make love to you. It is in those circumstances, that you are dependent on the therapist to recognize the difference between the feelings which you've artificially generated and which ones are real and to respect you sufficiently as an individual that he not mistreat you by misunderstanding what it is you are really expressing.

In the content there also will be times when the therapist will make interpretations which you won't like. You will think he's wrong and that anything that he says is wrong. He doesn't know what he's talking about and he doesn't understand you. Your feeling is that he's inept, stupid and totally wrong. Your initial reaction is your defensive system and may not be the end for that interpretation. Before you get into taking the action of walking out or cussing him out you ought to delay a little. Think it over. When I say "delay a little" it may take until the next session or the next two or three sessions before you actually make a judgment about whether what the therapist interpreted had any validity.

Therapists can be wrong and if the therapist is wrong you should be able to tell him on a direct basis that you disagree with him and that you think that what he told you did not have any bearing on what you were talking about or that it was inappropriate. Whatever it is, there should be verbal interchanges and no physical interchanges. The content of the therapy is basically what you bring to it. What you bring to it is not only the thoughts you have but also the feelings you have. Even though it may be a little difficult to accept or understand, the fact is that content includes feelings. Without those feelings the intellectual content has very little meaning. It's the feeling which gives meaning to the thoughts, the words, and the actions. Without those feelings there is no content.

Thinking only, without feeling, is sterile. It's unproductive.

Freud maintained that the royal road to the unconscious was through dreaming. Well, that may very well be true but at the same time that royal road to the unconscious is not the unconscious of the therapist but is the unconscious of the person having the dream. Any suggestion or characterization of the symbolism of the dreams by the therapist remains a product of the therapist's personality and not a product of the dreamer's personality. If you happen to be in treatment and trying to figure out what's going on so that you can reorganize your life and you begin having dreams, remember that it's up to you to let your fantasies go to interpret what that dream might mean to you. It doesn't really matter what your dream means to the therapist. The only thing that matters is what the dream means to you. Attempts to interpret dreams have gone on for eons. There are a great many references in the oldest of written languages of the meanings of dreams, in any culture.

In the past some psychiatrists have made long lists, including Freud by the way, of different forms, shapes, actions, as symbols and situations in a dream and interpreted those as though they were so many preconceived tables of meaning. A preconceived list or preconceived conceptualization of what all those indicators were in a dream as to what the dream might mean is futile. I feel that's all phony. What the dream might mean is what the dream means to you not what the dream means to the therapist. Any preconceived notion about a particular situation, or symbol, meaning a certain object or person or gender of a person in a dream is simply just not true. It can assume any kind of a transformation which the person who has the dream wants it to take or has going on in him. Dreams are a product of the mentation of the person having the dream.

There are many biblical references to the interpretations of dreams and what they might mean for the future and premonitions of what are things to come.

Those are all workings of the mind which mean that that individual has without knowing it, put together certain pieces of information, certain organizational systems within their own personality which add up to a prediction of something which is not necessarily going on now but is something which they can anticipate.

In the recent studies in research about dreaming it has been shown that dreams actually take place in a specific portion of the brain. That has always thought to be true but nobody has been able to demonstrate it. Now by special techniques of taking electrical samples of the brain cells in different areas of the brain and recording those as electroencephalograms. It has been shown that dreaming specifically correlates with a period of deep sleep called "REM" sleep, and occurs in the area of the brain known as the hippocampus.

What recent theorists have postulated is that the content of the dream is meaningless, as far as any symbolism is concerned and that the dreams represent an excessive amount of sensory reception during the previous few days or hours just prior to the night in which the person dreams. I am sure many psychiatrists will disagree with this opinion but the facts are that it is now possible to demonstrate that dreams do occur in specific areas of the brain and that those areas and the time of dreaming can be recorded by an electroencephalogram and that the content of the dream, then, is only what the dreamer determines it is. As yet there is no method to record the content of the dream, only the fact that it is occurring. Under these circumstances there is virtually no way that the therapist can suggest what the dream means and have it corroborated by the patient because what ever it is that the therapist suggests is bound to be a product of the therapist's mental functioning and not of the patient's.

On the other hand, some people who have premonitions of things that happen may arrange their lives without knowing it, to make that premonition come true so that it works both ways. It's almost as though the person is working toward that goal and that event without knowing that they are arranging it to happen. Then, having a dream only puts it into some kind of form which they can believe makes the premonition come true.

Also another kind of content has to do with horror dreams. Dreams in which the dreamer begins to feel that every dream is one of total disaster and that he is being engulfed by all kinds of monsters, situations, people and personalities that are very frightening and fearful. I think such dreams do represent the depth of your anxieties and your terrors but they can also be explained in part physiologically although what the physiological explanation is as of yet we really don't know.

Nonetheless, such dreams as nightmares which wake you up, don't have to be kinds of terror dreams. Sometimes nightmares are dreams of overt sexuality and if you are particularly fearful of the expression of overt sexuality that might be much of a nightmare to you and awaken you. The only difference between the definition of nightmares and an ordinary dream is that you wake up in terror.

It is not infrequent for people to wake up in the middle night and go back to sleep without any evidence of knowledge of dreaming or just remembering their dreams. The fact that a dream wakes you up and you are in terror is what makes it a nightmare. The fact that you just wake up and then go back to sleep doesn't make the dream a nightmare.

I also feel that many people have difficulties getting to sleep and staying asleep because they don't remember sleeping. It is the nature of sleep that we don't remember it. It is an activity by which we prepare ourselves for the next day's living and I have always looked upon it in that context.

Many people just lie in bed waiting for sleep to overcome them as though they had no activity or production in the manner in which they go to sleep or that they have no control over their sleep at all. It just happens to them. It seems to me that sleep is an activity just like playing baseball. In order to be able to get up and do what you need to do the following day and enjoy it, it's necessary to get your rest by sleeping. With this belief, I have never had any problems getting to sleep at night. I have felt that that sleep is a necessary activity for my existence and that if I wished to have a comfortable, pleasant and enthusiastic day the following day that I had better prepare for that day by getting my rest.

It is also true that not everybody sleeps well all the time. There are times when we all have our tensions and our anxieties put upon us and that these may become so great that at least for a few days or nights we have difficulty getting to sleep and when that happens, of course, it is frightening for the person to whom it happens. Such an episode of insomnia doesn't mean that it is necessary for you to get perturbed and begin to feel that you are having major problems with your mind.

Frequently, various physiological events may occur in your body that also cause you to have insomnia. Sometimes our dietary habits will cause insomnia and these are all topics which you should discuss with a physician in order that you will get some realistic basis for the reason you have difficulty in getting to sleep.

This kind of content is not something which many non physicians can discuss with you because the various effects of medications, drugs, condiments and other stimuli of that kind are usually not within the realm of their expertise and knowledge. In addition you don't tell them, even when they ask. But nonetheless too much coffee, tea, too many excesses of all kinds of things, especially alcohol if you are on any kind of psychotropic medication or if you use psychedelic drugs, such as marijuana, you are in for a hard time if you have insomnia because it is very difficult to pinpoint exactly what causes it. All of this, of course, is content for you to discuss in the interviews and make sure you talk with the therapist to let him know what your concerns are and what you have been doing to yourself. I feel very strongly that one of the biggest problems with being emotionally disturbed is reflected in the loss of sleep. If you don't get your rest at night it is very difficult for you to tackle the problems the next day. Sleeping is an absolute necessity for you to maintain yourself.

Whatever you do when you see a therapist don't try to plan what you are going to talk about before you get there. If you let it come out more spontaneously you will reach where you are going and what you are trying to do a lot more quickly.

You may try to plan a little bit if you have some difficulty with whatever medication you are on and you feel that it is troubling you. Then plan to talk with him about that. When it comes to any other content about what's going on within you, as far as your feelings are concerned, the more you plan it the more you are likely to disrupt the very purpose for your being there and make it much more difficult for him to meet your needs and make the relationship between you real. Planning what to talk about is a way of avoiding expressing your feelings.

The key to most therapy is spontaneity and you do need to have intellectual and emotional spontaneity to be effective even though to you it will seem that you are going extremely slow. If you are preoccupied with things that are going on during the day, with your work, just talk about whatever comes up that's what Freud meant by "free association".

The more you try to plan what you are going to talk about the less effective you will be. Planning what to talk about only constitutes a protectionism built within you so that you do not hear those things about yourself that you do not want to hear. Planning what you are going to talk about is a defense dynamism which protects you from the spontaneity of your own feelings and of the interrelationship between you and the therapist and impedes the progress of your treatment rather than aids it.

One of the concepts I have about treatment, which is not original with me, is that you are not being honest with yourself about what it is you're expressing. (Helmut Kaiser) All of us have in us those very primitive feelings of anger, hostility, affection, fear and terror with which everyone is equipped. What makes the difference is whether or not we are honest with ourselves in the expression of them and especially allowing ourselves to recognize that we have those feelings. (Hamlet Act I Scene 3) Society does not permit us to totally express hostile feelings and kill some one. For that we go to jail and sometimes are put to death. The other extreme of making love with someone in public is also unacceptable and we can go to jail for that too. We need to express our feelings within the acceptable social limits which are not written down. Only those acts which are not acceptable are prohibited by law.

None of us loves everybody. None of us hates everybody. It is perfectly legitimate to have feelings of mild hostility and antagonism towards some person and to also have feelings of affection for them. But what makes a difference in our getting along and in treatment, is how we manifest those feelings in the course of the interview.

    We can believe and think and feel anything we like. What we do is what makes a difference in getting into social difficulties. Thinking is private, just within ourselves if we keep it there. Action is public. Any and everyone else can either observe or conclude we have taken some action and that's when the problems begin.

Kaiser, Helmut   The Contributions of Helmut Kaiser
                     Effective Psychotherapy
    Ed. : Louis B. Fierman, M.D.; Allen J. Enlow, M.D.
       The Free Press, New York, 1965

Shakespeare, William The Tragedy of Hamlet
                    Prince of Denmark
              Act I, Scene 3

CHAPTER 10

Whether or not any physical contact, i.e., touch, should occur between two people who are in a therapeutic session, under any circumstances, has been a very controversial discussion for many years.

Since touch is one of the most primitive of our sensations and can note a very wide variety of expressions of feeling, of the full gamut of feelings, is the very reason for the controversy which exists about touching during therapy.

There are times when there is either inadvertent or purposeful touch in the casual course of human conversation. There are times when touch of course, represents the most aggressive of our emotional outbursts and there are other times when it can represent the most affectionate feelings. The skin, which is the largest organ in the body, is also the most sensuous.

To make the distinction between appropriateness or inappropriateness, when touch occurs, is a difficult decision.

For example, if on a cold day, a lady is putting on her coat after a session, prior to going out into the cold, the therapist as common courtesy, should try to assist her getting into her coat, it is very likely the therapist would be touching her in some form by simply holding the coat out for her to slip her arms in the arm holes. There are people who feel that even that is an unacceptable form of touch from a therapist.

There are other times when in the expression of deep grieving for something which has occurred, either in the present or the past, that some form of comfort by laying on of hands, such as a hug, from the therapist onto you, may be more relieving of that sense of loss for you than anything else that can occur. A simple holding of the hands is an expression of empathy (I can appreciate how you feel. I've had the same feeling) that the therapist can convey an acceptance of the emotional pain which you are having. Holding hands is not always a sexual experience.

On the other hand, violent physical contact, such as slapping you or you slapping the therapist in the heat of anger, when you may feel that the therapist has said something or interpreted something which you feel is grossly inappropriate, even though no previous touch had occurred, may be the expression of the violent anger and hatred of that particular moment on your part or on the part of the therapist, whoever does the slapping.

All of these forms are representative extremes and of course, the one extreme which is talked about the most is the therapist "taking advantage" of you by offering sexual comforts to you, presumably to relieve your grief over the loss or inadequacies of affection for sexual needs. Of course this latter is what is talked about the most. It is also true in some instances, that you may entice the therapist into having some kind of affectionate touch between you. It makes no difference whether you are female and the therapist is male or whether you are male and the therapist is female or whether you are both the same sex. Affection can be expressed in this kind of a touching situation and it is always interpreted as being the responsibility of the therapist to see that it does not occur and to halt the process of therapy at that point as such physical sexual contacts are not considered to be therapeutic.

On the other hand, there are some organizations which are specifically organized by therapist's who say they really believe that sexual contact between the therapist and the patient is not only permissible, but it is a positive therapeutic experience for the patient. There continues to be a great deal of controversy about this concept and behavior. A great majority of therapists do not accept the view that sexual contact is therapeutic and a great majority of therapists feel that any sexual contact or direct sexual stimulation between the therapist and the patient is always inappropriate. Most of the women to whom this happens also feel that it is not appropriate, and that their trust in the therapist, as well as their bodies, had been violated.

Some studies have shown, or at least reported to have shown, that sexual contacts between the therapist and patient occurs a lot more frequently than is commonly thought. Hugs have been defined as sexual contacts for some of such studies. Most people would define kissing, or intercourse as sexual contacts, but not necessarily hugs. Stroking breasts, or genitals I feel is also sexual contact, but not necessarily hugs. A great proportion of such studies refer to the male therapist and the female patient.

On the other hand, physical contact, such as hugs, may or may not be a sexual assault or suggestion. It may be a very comforting thing to you. It does not make any difference what your sex or the sex of the therapist is.

In some circumstances, when you are in the deep throes of emotional reliving of previous experiences, you are relating to the therapist as though you are a child and under these circumstances to treat you as a child and ignore your physically adult body is appropriate because at that moment, emotionally, both of you are children. It is quite appropriate to give you the emotional response which you wanted to have as a child, including hugs.

In some cultures, a kiss on the cheek is a form of greeting. It is not considered to be a sexual assault or a sexual invitation. But, in our culture a kiss on the cheek is usually reserved for the closest family relatives. It is true in many cultures, especially in the European cultures, that the formalized "kiss on both cheeks", represents a form of greeting and a salutation without any sexual connotation of any kind, but basically a respect for the individual, regardless of the sexes of the people involved. These kinds of ceremonial kisses and ceremonial hugs are completely acceptable most of the time. There is absolutely no reason why they should not occur in private when they are simply ceremonial hugs or ceremonial kisses on the cheek, or pats on the back or head. Not pats on the buttocks.

None the less, the physical aspects of touch between a patient and the therapist have always remained a very controversial topic. I was quite surprised when I learned in some research, that some of the researchers considered "hugs" to be a sexual assault on the patient. There are times when that kind of a physical touch with the patient is the most reassuring, the least stimulating and the most satisfying feeling of acceptance from the patient or the therapist. A mutual sharing of that experience with no sexual connotation of any kind. At that point in the exchange both you and the therapist are emotional children.

Some of our television personalities, such as Leo Bastoglia, advocate the expression of love between people. By this, he does not mean they should have sexual relations in the middle of the street, but that the physical contact of shaking hands, hugging, kissing one another on the cheeks, sharing the touching experiences in public are all expressions of love and that it should be promoted and that it does more good than harm to share these kinds of expressions of affection which are not sexual in connotation, depending on the feelings between the participants.

The question arises about what the motivation is for these feelings. If this is to share love, but it is in private, then there are a lot of people who feel that the therapeutic relationship from a professional to a laymen, a hug is inappropriate.

I do not agree. I feel that it is perfectly appropriate, depending on the circumstances and what your and the therapist's emotional feelings are at that time. To give some one a hug, a pat on the back or to dry their tears with a facial tissue without making any such experience a sexual assault, or suggestion, can be a sharing of emotionality and nothing else, not a sexual invitation or sexual provocation.

Whether such physical contacts between the therapist and the patient that do become sexual or aggressive, in large measure is dependent on the emotional stability and maturity of the individuals involved, especially the therapist.

In this respect, the emotional maturity of the therapist is something which must be at high level for these kinds of touches to be effective and therapeutic. Unfortunately, not all therapists are emotionally that mature. There are therapists who do "try to take advantage" of their patients or clients, for their own personal emotional satisfaction and exploit the patients who may be vulnerable to such personal contacts.

It is necessary to remember that therapy is an emotional experience in and of itself. The purpose of therapy is to help you become more aware, feel more satisfaction, to find new ways of expressing your emotions and your feelings. The continued use of the methods of expression which you had developed are less effective than they were in the past. It is the failure of the expression of your emotional feelings and sensations, whether they be aggressive or affectionate, that brings you into the therapist in the first place.

It is the failure of communication from one person to another which causes you to seek treatment in the first place. In your failure to communicate and to be able to express and receive emotional feelings adequately and accurately between you and other individuals. It is necessary for you to experience those feelings and to find that you are safe and you can express your feelings in ways different from the manner which you were using prior to your therapeutic experience. All such changes in our way of doing things are very slow to come about even if we are accustomed to break the ice by needing a cocktail or two. It should not be necessary for anyone to have alcohol in order to converse with someone else. On the other hand, some people are embarrassed and feel awkward balancing teacups at a tea party and such people find it difficult to break the barrier to say "I'm Mary Smith" or "I'm Harry Jones" to break the ice, although on a one to one basis once you get through that initial awkwardness you may be a very warm individual.

Since touch is such a primitive communication system and does convey feelings so effectively, it can be an important method of finding that bridge between people, when otherwise the bridge may be very tenuous. A handshake is touch.

What the effect of touch is during the course of therapeutic contact, is largely dependent on the emotional maturity of the therapist and the emotional needs of the so called patient.

However, in my opinion, there is no justification for direct sexual stimulation resulting from touch, even though it may be a mutually pleasurable experience at the time, I think it is devastating for treatment. I suggest that in the event you feel that the touching that is going on during the course of the treatment may be leading to some kind of sexual intimacies, I recommend that you pick up your hat, your purse, your coat, briefcase or whatever else you are carrying, and leave.

Touch is a sensual experience, like sex, but it should be confined to touch and not expanded to sex.

Some of the social situations in which you find yourself are going to include those circumstances in which alcohol is being served. It is a fact that alcohol and psychotropic medications of various kinds, especially the antianxiety drugs and the major neuroleptic medications, are simply not compatible. What happens is that the medication gives the alcohol an effect three or four times greater than it would have if you were not on medication. Just stopping your medication for one or two doses before you go to a party will not be effective because there will still be enough medication in your body to react with alcohol and will still have that enhanced effect.

Of course you know, if you are going to try to protect yourself from letting other people know you are going to a psychiatrist then drinking anything is likely to let the cat out of the bag. Alcohol loosens the barriers of social control and can enhance sensation so it is dangerous beyond an specified intake level. That intake point is different for each individual. Beyond that point thinking processes become damaged and not reliable.

If you are progressing at all and coming to find yourself getting more self confidence, never mind what other people think. It doesn't make any difference if you want to hold a glass to prevent having to answer too many questions. Get some non intoxicating beverage, any of the soft drinks, and you can stand around with that in your hand and no one can tell the difference anyway. You might know it but no one else will.

The likelihood of your spilling the beans and being more embarrassed at such a party is considerably better if you have even one drink so I think the behavior that is the least likely to let everybody know that you are seeing a psychiatrist is to drink nothing that has alcohol in it.

In some instances if you want to get a little high you might take some ice tea or iced coffee and even if it's diluted or decaffeinated. You're going to have some kind of a little boost from the fluid whether the caffeine and the theobromine is in the tea or not. That might make you feel a little more confidant rather than just drinking some soft drink .

In all circumstances in a social situation, at least in the beginning, what you need to keep on your mind is that you are the equal of anyone else. They are there just like you are in order to be seen and maybe to discuss some of the issues of the day or the issues of what that meeting is about. Small talk is the order of the day so if you can let yourself feel confident you can talk with them about anything. You will gain self confidence as you go and such kinds of social encounters are a very distinct asset rather than a liability.

However, I am sure the first time you go to one of those gatherings you will be scared to death and you will believe that everyone there knows all about you. You will probably be shaking inside. Your palms may be sweating but if you do it, getting through it will give you the confidence that you can do it again. Each time you do it will become easier and of course you will be gaining self confidence by leaps and bounds. As you do and by the time you have gone to half a dozen such gatherings you will feel a lot more comfortable than you did to start with. You might even come to enjoy them.

Always remember if you meet your psychiatrist or your therapist that they are people too and that's all. When you are out in a circumstance like that they are no better or different from you and really don't carry anymore weight than you do as far as the overall party conditions are concerned.

It is out in those social gatherings where you may also be most exposed to the influence of touch. Some people touch more easily after they have had a cocktail or two. They either get belligerent or they get affectionate. These same people usually react the same way at different parties as their reactions are a function of their personalities. Your reactions are also a function of your personality and you will respond with either a snarl or feelings of conviviality and affection. Sexually aroused feelings may also occur, whether it be with the therapist or someone else. It is at these times when the therapist personal emotional strength will be measured. If the therapist becomes affectionate then your strength will be measured as it will be evident that the therapist had already lost control.

It will be an "eye opener" for you to see your therapist in circumstances which you did not expect and probably never imagined. Your reaction to the revelation about the therapist might well be an important recognition of the frailty of the therapist and your strength of character to provide an even greater lift to your self appraisal.

It is possible that your inflated appraisal of the therapist personality might burst and leave you with a quite detrimental, revised estimate of your former idol. It will be proof that therapists are only people with all the human frailties. It could benefit you a great deal to continue to go to that therapist for your change in adjustment to exercise your new found emotional strength.

CHAPTER 11

The pleasure we derive in life often comes in the struggle. Struggle comes in three major types- physical, intellectual and emotional. Some people would also say financial. If the first three are successful the financial will follow.

When we set goals in life for ourselves and make a plan, if we think, we tackle the world with all the biological force we can bring to bear to achieve those goals. In olden times our wants were more simply satisfied, not less complex but we were satisfied with adequate lodging,(a roof, some heat and protection from the weather) food and companionship even though we probably did not understand the whys and wherefors as to why we wanted them. We only knew and felt more comfortable with them. It took a great deal more physical effort to get those basics for both men and women, and because of the hazards of everyday life from the elements and predators, life was not so long as it is now.

Over the years our needs haven't changed but our desires ("would like to haves") have changed. In order to achieve a tighter roof, running water, electric lights and appliances, and, or natural gas or electricity for heating, cooling and cooking, man has developed an increasingly technological world which takes less direct physical effort to use, at least for the person who turns on the switch, strikes the match, or pushes the button on the pieza electric crystal to start the flame. Now, various kinds of sensors may do it "automatically" with our doing nothing more than speaking, walking into a room, shutting the door or leaving the room or opening the door. The same energy, and perhaps more energy, to achieve the same satisfaction is used, only it is not so direct. It is more hidden from our direct sensation as other people who contribute to our comfort are miles away from us performing the myriad of complex tasks which are required in consort, to achieve what seems to an "effortless" activity. Our ancestors didn't have to worry about getting exercise to keep their hearts and lungs in good physical shape. Their lives were exercise to keep alive.

Over the years our needs haven't changed but our desires have. As man achieved increased technology it is apparent that our desires have increased along with the complexity of technology.

The physical energy which we put forth using our own muscles has decreased to a considerable extent. Technology has reduced the necessity for personal physical energy. Now most people need to get exercise in order to keep their bodies fit. There are many occupations in which this is not necessary but at the same time the majority of occupations are far more sedentary than they were in the past. For example, it was not necessary for a farmer or even the earliest planters to seek exercise in order to keep their bodies fit. Their problem was finding enough food to keep their bodies healthy enough to perform the exercise. The simplest gardeners planted their crops by making a hole in the ground with a stick, putting the seed in and waiting, hopefully, for the rain to come.

Now, farmers work most of their crops with tractors and many other pieces of complex machinery which they use as well as fertilizer in order the get the maximum crop. They also irrigate. Irrigation has been used for thousands of years. Some places in the "New World" of South and Central America are now known to have been irrigated as much as three thousand years ago and probably much longer in the Mediterranean Basin and in the Orient. Now, farmers raise thousands of times more than they themselves need and that is converted into money with which they are able to obtain the necessities which they need. At least in the United States they raise thousands of times more than they themselves need. Other countries may not be so fruitful and many must import food for their population.

In the cities, the situation has become desperate where there are now so many people it is impossible for them to revert to the more primitive practice of growing their own food because it is impossible to grow crops in concrete. Nor can plants and animals survive on concrete. Food has to be provided for them. It is impossible for them to scrounge for themselves in the natural food chain in order to survive. The tensions and anxieties of more primitive peoples were just as real to them as our tensions are real to us today. Additional sources of tension and anxiety are what is commonly referred to as "stress" are now due to more multiple causes than they were previously. Just having the basic needs now is not enough. Stresses often come up between people and particularly in families. Everyday living to meet the expenses of the household as well as having money left over for what we consider pleasure creates "stress", conflict between members of the family.

This puts a burden on the younger individuals because now a great deal more education is required to survive and be competitive in the world different from what was needed to be competitive in previous times.

It makes no difference what type of work the breadwinner goes into. It is true, that it is generally conceded that greater education is now required in order to be a successful competitor even if one wants to be a farmer.

That seems to be one of the problems of the so called "lower classes". The lower classes are not just lower because they live in less affluent circumstances, in part they live in less affluent circumstances because they are less well educated. However, in general they get more exercise. As one becomes more educated one generally obtains a more sedentary job. It makes little difference into which intellectual area of activity one achieves there is less physical effort, with some exceptions. The performing arts, such as music, dancing, acting, sports as well as others are notable exceptions. It takes considerable intellectual struggle to master and memorize the scores, routines and skills. It also takes a great deal of physical effort to perform the total body control which is necessary to make the presentation. Even singing requires a large lung capacity as well as the control of vocal cords to produce the sounds. Another area is professional athletics of various kinds.

For you as a person to try to meet this challenge once you become an adult is considerably more difficult. Without an education, once a family is started, the routine living expenses seem to take up most of the family income and time. Changing directions of trying to become better educated to make a better income becomes much more difficult.

It is true that not all sources of income, depending on the activity, are directly dependent on the quantity or the quality of education that one receives. There are some activities to which some people aspire, such as the arts of various kinds, professional athletics as well as others, in which individuals seem to be very successful in spite of having not pursued nor accomplished much formal academics. Their education in training their bodies or their minds to perform takes a great deal more time than the majority of people seem to recognize. Furthermore, in order for them to be successful in maintaining themselves after they have come to the end of their productive lives means that many of them have had to earn that living for the total span of years of their lives in many fewer years.

Successfully competing bodies seem to lose their winning edge faster than do successfully competing minds. On the other hand, physically healthy bodies are necessary for comfort and aid in prolonging a more pleasant existence and a healthy mind.

When your stress gets high you have to take a look at yourself to figure out whether or not you can change directions to different ways of earning an income or whether by pursuing what you have already started you can successfully compete during your older years.

The pleasure which we receive in the struggle doesn't seem to be such a pleasure at the time we are going through it, particularly when it begins very young. It is all work. There should be at least some formal intellectual education during the time the body is being trained to be successfully competitive .

In intellectual activity as a means of earning a living, the struggle takes a different form in that intellectual learning may be more prolonged than the physical activity required to prepare one for the use of one's body in the competition of earning a living.

None of these activities comes cheaply. There isn't any way I know that anybody can make some achievements to reach their goals except by effort.

The only way I know is to inherit it and fortunately none of us picks out our ancestors. We don't have the choice of selecting the root from which we are derived and what ever impinges on us from our biological roots we are stuck with, good and bad.

That means that our particular genes may give us some unusual configuration of body appearance. They may give us some unusual metabolism. They may give us some unusual color, hormonal balance or configuration which may not be quite as acceptable in society. The social and cultural mores may impinge on us and all of those require an adjustment if one is to achieve some goals in living. No one knows how much of our intellectual capacity is genetically determined.

Unfortunately, a great many people really don't set any particular goals for themselves. They go through life just trying to absorb whatever pleasures they can and use their energies in the pursuit of pleasure for itself with the result that many of them expect someone else to care for them when the going gets tough and they fall victim to a physical injury or disease, or a mental disease which makes the adjustment harder or forces them to turn to a new system of life to survive. Some are not able to make the adjustment which is necessary in order to be a successful competitor. Often what are pursued as "pleasures" when one is young are the cause of premature failure as we age. Alcohol is the prime example. Smoking is another example.

Fortunately, some are able to make a new start in life when such disasters occur. I have known men who had always earned a living for their families by using their muscles in laboring work because they had not the confidence in themselves to believe that they were able to achieve an advanced academic education to earn a living by thinking. After serious accidents or illnesses which left them physically incapacitated they were able to start over to go to high school or college to obtain degrees in an activity which did not require major physical effort. They were able to educate themselves to earn a living with their minds rather than with their muscles. As they went through the struggle to get to class on time and to train themselves to use their minds to learn different kinds of knowledge the struggle was heroic but if it had not been for the "disaster" of having had the injury they would never had the courage to try and to believe that they could make the effort to succeed in mental activity. Sometimes what seems to be a total loss in life turns out to be a blessing in disguise since it forced them to change their way of life or not be competitive. Having made the struggle, when they look back on themselves and realize that they had changed their entire attitude about themselves and their way of life they are only remorseful that they had not had the courage to do it sooner. They are also very thankful that they had succeeded in changing and often found themselves in a more lucrative life style than they would had had in the long run if they had not changed.

One man I remember had been a truck driver with a wife and two children. He had been involved in an accident and fire which was not of his making. He survived, and in surviving lost both his legs above the knees. He went to school, became educated and became a manager of the company for which he had worked as a truck driver. Although he had many physical limitations as a result of having lost his legs, he had a more satisfying life with his wife and children than he had had before. It was a massive struggle for the entire family, not just for him, and in the process they almost lost each other because of the fear of his inability to earn a living for them. In the process his wife learned that she was capable of earning money on which to live, but she also learned that she, too, would have to have more education if she were to earn as much as he had earned as a truck driver. She also learned that she really did not want to work in the commercial world. She was much more content to stay at home with the children to raise and educate rather than having to compete outside the home. In the long run one might say that the entire family, each individual, benefited because he lost his legs. That only came about because together they undertook a massive struggle from which they could not know in advance whether or not they could be successful.

Struggle also comes with events which may not incapacitate, such as with deaths of people in the family of whom we are fond, having to make adjustments to new neighbors, having to move to another city because of transfers or finding a new job. Any change that comes to us when we are settled into our daily rut of living is a struggle to master. Life itself is a continuous change.

The emotional struggle to survive is just as real as the physical and intellectual and requires the successful application of both the other two types. Anxiety has been described as our protective emotional system, until it gets to be too strong then it becomes a detriment. On the other hand "over educated fools" who never take a good look at the world around them, nor adapt to the demands the world makes on them, are just as likely to fail as other inept people. Certainly, unless the highly paid professional athletes make provision for their after peak physical years they, too, will fail. Adaptation is a constant requirement. Intellectual types have to find ways of keeping their bodies physically fit or they, too, fail. Anxiety is the glue which keeps people on the road to adaptation regardless of their circumstances.

Other emotional reactions such as depression, aggression, insomnia, physical ailments, aches, pains, all may be the product of our collective biological systems telling us that we need to reassess ourselves to find out what we are doing to ourselves. In order to make that reassessment we must struggle with our intellectual and emotional systems to take a look at ourselves differently from the automatic system we had developed while we were maturing. That takes a tremendous amount of struggle as it takes much energy to study ourselves to combat the automatisms of adaptations which we had developed and which at one time in our lives had served us well.

The fact that you are seeking help in reassessing yourself is a partial product of the struggle within you which has already occurred. You have won this first struggle to change and now you are embarking on the change itself.

CHAPTER 12

In our every day living we react emotionally, and our bodies react physically, at various physiological levels of which some are extremely primitive and of which we are almost never aware.

The autonomic nervous system, for example, which regulates the activity of our intestines, blood vessels and other internal organs is so automatic that none of us ever feels, in any true sense, digestion of food or movement of food through the intestines. Our hormonal systems are also so automatic that what we feel are the results of the interplay of our hormones. The hormones themselves are not felt in any conscious manner. A classic example are the variations of the hormonal levels in the life of a woman, in which she has periodic menstrual cycles and maybe moods in accordance with the shifts of the levels of concentration of hormones within her body, over which she has absolutely no conscious control. Men, ordinarily, do not have any sensation of shifts of their moods, or insofar as anyone knows, major periodic shifts of their hormonal levels during the course of their life span. Hormones come from hormone glands, pituitary, adrenal, pancreas, thyroid and many others. Men's reproductive hormones are not so obviously cyclical as women's. They produce sperm 24 hours a day, every day, until that capacity is lost for life.

On the other hand, men are also subject to mood changes; they are subject to some hormonal changes, even though these are not well known but operate 24 hours a day, 7 days a week, from the time before we are born until we die. There are many hormones which are common to both sexes, all of which function constantly. The constancy or inconstancy of hormonal shifts and changes occur with our nutritional state because hormones are dependent on an adequate and proper balance of nutritional intake of all known types of food and "trace elements", which are substances in very small amounts in our body necessary to produce the physiological balances of life. Trace elements are metallic elements which are an integral part of hormones, enzymes, proteins and complex lipoproteins as well as many other compounds in the body. Their presence is a requirement to facilitate the metabolic processes which are normal physiological functions. For example, recently it has been discovered that unless magnesium is present that post menopausal women can not make use of adequate supplies of calcium and female hormones to maintain proper bone strength and prevent osteoporosis. It has also been demonstrated, with women, that those who suffer with osteoporosis can be made healthy again when adequate supplies of magnesium, estrogens, and calcium are all supplied. The magnesium seems to act as a catalyst and produces more enzymes to permit new bone to be formed and strengthen the old bone. This process takes several years to perform- just as it takes several years for the bone to deteriorate when there is not enough magnesium, female hormones, and calcium.

Of course, vitamins are the other essential "trace" substances which are necessary for adequate functioning. Without them our bodies are just as vulnerable to disturbances as without the trace elements. We have known about vitamin deficiencies for a much longer period of time than the trace metallic elements. We have also known about poisoning from too much of some kinds of vitamins as well as poisoning from too strong a concentration of the heavy metals, true poisons. The same trace metals which are considered poisons are also necessary in their normal concentration for proper nutrition. Any substance can become a poison when it is abused. Either too much or too little. Water, either in excess or depletion becomes dangerous and deadly.

At a more complex, abstract, "higher" level of organization in our body in the sense that we are more aware of it. We may believe that we are "thinking" as though that were some kind of an abstract function over which we have some control.

The facts are, we have very little control over our thinking. Only as we lead ourselves from one "thought" to another by some mysterious means which we call "association". Of course various memories may come back to us and become conscious when they reach a critical level of intensity. We don't know what constitutes a "critical" level of intensity to make the memory conscious.

On the other hand, no one knows what constitutes a memory or how a memory is retained physiologically, nor what the intensity is which is necessary for that memory to become conscious, and we become aware that we are having it. There are many memories and associations which are completely outside of our awareness Nonetheless, they are very real and are the processes on which we act.

The more primitive level of adjustment is action, muscle action. I wrote in chapter five that I don't like to get hit by a patient, but I don't mind them being angry with me. I don't mind getting kissed, on the cheek, by a patient because that helps both of us feel "warm" toward each other. Getting hit makes us feel "cold" or " hot", both angry, toward each other. These are simple levels of very primitive reaction patterns which go on in a person and which a person may use as a routine adaptation to living, whether he is aware of it or not. They are aware of the result but not always aware of the thought to do it. The action frequently comes faster than the thought.

I think of different types of people as being "action oriented" in that they express their feelings by actions rather than thinking first and then acting or self containment of trying to delay the impulses they feel to take action.

Impulsivity is the inability to delay the action which occurs, and it usually occurs prior to any thought about what is going on. One simply reacts with totality and then kind of "explodes" in some kind of action, usually it's physical in nature, striking, hitting, running, jumping, leaving and maybe even fainting or having a seizure.

When it comes to seizures, we have to also discriminate between seizures of physical losses of control and social losses of control. Physical losses of control is loss of control in which the muscles contract; we lose control over our bowels and maybe bite our tongue, lose control over our urinary functions. Social losses of control occur when the social situation is inappropriate for the particular muscle action we take.

It might be that an action, for example, of being very disruptive in classrooms or being too loud, inappropriate activity and so on. It may be the expression of a kind of "social seizure" which might be very deeply rooted and at the same basic physiological level as a physical seizure in which the muscles contract. A so called temper tantrum.

Such outbursts of temper, of affection, of physical seizures, grinding our teeth, thumbing our nose, fondling our hair, picking our nose all become manifestations of some portions of our personality. Any such manifestations are lumped together to give everyone a mental picture and definition of emotion.

We define our emotions by our physiological reactions. Different emotions are made up of many of the same kinds of physiological reactions and the complex of physiological reactions defines our emotions. That particular emotion is named by the thoughts which go along with it in a particular episode. For example, blood pressure goes up in anger and in love making and we are not aware of it. We call it love making or anger, not high blood pressure. We only call it high blood pressure when there are no particular thoughts or feelings associated with it.

Anxiety, fear and terror are degrees of the same physiological complexes. Our automatic body functions differ in the degree of strength of their reactions but we label them in accordance with our mental set at the time. They are our emotions. Depression, mania, love, anger are interpreted by our mind differently and our "mind" is an indefinable (as yet) set of such interactions, many of which we are now getting better able to define in neurotransmitter or neurophysiological terms. Certainly, this science is very primitive but psychiatrists and neurophysiologists are making steady, but irregular progress toward a much better understanding about what happens. There may come a time when the social manifestations of our emotional expressions and actions will be referred to by their neurophysiological terms and neurotransmitter sequences, or simultaneous functions.

None of the enzymes, chemical transmitters, or hormones is ever totally in command, nor totally depleted as any such system or function must be in some sort of balance or we die. We cannot survive when extremely out of physiological balance.

However, the malfunction of one set of these processes can be so severe that it causes something else to malfunction and we develop serious complications with major physical disease. Should our blood pressure go so high during a fit of anger that the blood vessels cannot withstand the pressure created and either rupture, or "blow out" with an aneurysm we could have a stroke or a serious hemorrhage to threaten or end our life.

Research scientists from all walks of biological sciences are busy trying to unravel what all the relationships are amongst all the substances, and their metabolism in order to create new drugs and methods of treatment. It has been only in the past three or four decades that sufficient technological advances have been made to study these events. Biological sciences are dependent on the advances made in physical sciences to do research. Some drugs to treat the mind can be made artificially and portions of them manipulated to create new drugs with new effects. As yet, there are very few drugs which act only on one organ or cell type which are being tried. There are practically none of them on the shelves because the science is too new and testing methods are to crude to establish the effects, and to see how they effect the person and personality in the various organ systems. Scientists also have to find out how new drugs interact with other drugs as two drugs may have reactions totally different from the reaction either drug alone creates.

Any drug we take has many more than one effect. They affect the whole body, wherever in the body the particular cells or other chemicals on which they act are present. Nonetheless, what they do in their primary, major action, is the basis for prescribing. Sometimes after several years, what were thought to be secondary, or side effects, become the indication for their use and the first primary indication for their use becomes the secondary one. There are always many such side effects, some of which are more a nuisance than a help. Sometimes in different people the side effects so disturb the person that it is necessary to abandon that drug and try another drug. It is not infrequent that several drugs have to be tried before one is found which performs as it is designed to, without the serious side effects, in that person.

It is difficult for many people for whom drugs are prescribed to accept the fact that the medication which the physician chooses behaves so badly that it can't be used. Many people begin to believe that the physician who had made the prescription is not a good physician. Such an occurrence does not make him a poor physician. He just had the bad luck to select a drug which does not work well with that particular person.

Another problem which arises is that different drugs prescribed for a particular symptom may be a perfectly good drug but in the presence of other drugs in the body the two drugs interact with each other and may create major imbalances. Often, it is not possible to predict how two drugs will interact as that information may not be available. No one may know, in spite of the extensive effort to find out prior to releasing the drug for general consumption. Should the drug be withheld from the public until all such information were available it could take decades to try all the experiments necessary to establish those facts. New drugs coming to the public would be few and far between and would be so expensive that no one could afford them. The price paid for a drug has to pay for all the research which went into it to develop it for use. The opposite of that is that if drugs were not reasonably tested they might be exceedingly dangerous, and perhaps deadly.

"Normal" physiological functions in the body vary a great deal within one person and from person to person with the result that the kind of medication one person is able to take successfully may not be compatible with another person. Physiology is not known for any absolutes. All processes may be slightly different from one person to another.

What happens to you physiologically is peculiar to you. Like finger prints, exact copies of physiological processes are very rare. Even the genetic structure of identical twins may not be exactly identical, nor will their physiological processes be exactly identical. There are wide variations of educated guesses in the field of "genetic printing" as to the frequency of repetition of what is now called "genetic finger prints". Ratios vary from 1:500,00 to 1:2,500,000 and no one knows the exact answer. So, too, may your physiological processes vary from every one else's. Certainly your personality varies from everyone else's. Your personality is the totality of your physiological processes. We have not yet come to the stage at which we can define personality as an mathematical expression of ratios of the known neurotransmitters in relation to each other. But, the time will come.

Medication and psychotherapy alter your physiological processes. The use of medication is more predictable than the use of another person's personality to modify your physiological processes, (your personality) because with medication, we are being exposed to the same, known, chemical formula whereas in psychotherapy the formula of the therapist's personality cannot be so well defined. In addition to which, the formula for the therapist's personality may change from session to session which further complicates the situation between the "patient" and the "therapist". There is little predictability from session to session.

As I noted previously, many people fear medications because of the possibility of becoming "hooked", addicted, to them as though there were no possibility of becoming addicted to psychotherapy. The likelihood of getting too dependent on the therapist is very real. Such dependency may be more devastating to making an adjustment in the real world than addiction to a medication.

"Orthodox" psychoanalysts depend on what they call "the transference neurosis" for the therapeutic effect which creates the cure, relieving the neurosis. Such a relationship between the patient and therapist is an addiction to the therapist in the form of the personality pattern of the patient from which it is hoped the patient may become conscious of what that relationship is, as expressed in terms of the significant figures of the past. What such "insight" does is reawaken the presumed relationships which are expressed in terms of significant figures or events of the past.

There is no guarantee that what is "remembered" was an event or only a fantasy and called a memory. What such a tortuous, time consuming chain of events does is lend some believed credence to what are called memories, which may or may not be true. It does nothing to actually change the concurrent neurophysiological events which I am calling personality. To change the neurophysiological chain of events remains another problem, and if those events gather some strength in a transference neurosis they are that much more difficult to change. The patient has become addicted to the therapist and the therapist has ensured himself of a reasonably secure income for the near future. The patient or client has achieved an addiction similar to that of the physical addiction brought on by ingested or incorporated chemicals, including medication.

In spite of all the complexities and difficulties which I depicted above, it is within your capabilities to do all this yourself. You can change your own neurophysiological personality by self examination. I do not mean that it is easy, but by being honest with yourself you can conduct your own examination and in the process of being honest with yourself alter the automatic responses which you had developed over your years of living.

You do that by imposing a delay in yourself in taking action. By asking yourself if you are interpreting accurately what you believe is going on around you in your communication with others or what your initial impression is.

If you ask yourself how else may what I see be interpreted ? Am I receiving those signals from outside with the same meaning in which they are sent ? Or is it possible that the other person means something other than my initial impression ? Also ask yourself, am I sending the signals I am trying to send ? How is the other person receiving what I am trying to convey ? By the simple act of delaying your response you are at the same time disrupting the automatic neurophysiological chains within yourself. Those chains by which you take action - the action of speaking, shrugging, throwing a fist, or hugging. In so delaying your response you can activate a new set of neurophysiological events within yourself and gradually change your personality. Then you may find yourself going into an entirely new direction by activating the new channels of nervous energy. You are changing yourself.

You may or may not feel anything physical within yourself except perhaps some sense of confusion such as what do I do now ? What happens next ? I have never done this before and I am in strange territory because it is a new experience and I feel lost because it doesn't feel familiar. I have no data base of experience which comes into automatic operation and I have to feel my way along to see what comes next or what I think or do next. You will probably feel quite anxious because you will not be able to predict exactly what will happen next and that in itself is frightening and thus anxiety producing.

Anxiety is also a set of neurophysiological reactions and you may find yourself sweating, shaking, puzzled or your hair might "stand on end". The first few times you try to delay action for such a self examination, you possibly will feel as though you are having a panic reaction. Should you just let your body react without applying some brain action in thinking you will be in a panic attack and may lose that episode for constructive purposes. Should you just let your panic attack take over you will be setting up a new pathway for panic attacks to occur more easily in the future and the experience may be more detrimental than helpful. The next time the anxiety will or may appear more easily and you will have taken a step backwards but with a new neurophysiological chain of events.

Nothing is easy. No change comes without effort and in such an instance as I describe it will be emotionally painful. Unless you are willing to withstand the sensations of anxiety, and emotional pain you are not likely to make much progress for this particular time.

As you gain more experience with these kinds of chains of events they will become less frightening and will be a signal that you have done something new rather than just proceeded down the same old path and gotten back into your old way of reacting. With enough experience the anxiety will decrease and you will adopt the new way of reacting more automatically and it will become the data base for a new way of examining yourself more impartially and more effectively. In a sense, one part of you will be like a referee, sitting back and examining what you are doing at the same time you are doing it and feeling the pleasure of doing it.

All such changes occur in small increments. It is not very likely that any major shifts in your personality will occur suddenly, or in huge strides. However, as the small changes do occur they have an indirect influence on future incidents, and they may lead to major, more satisfactory changes in your life style and sense of well being and self esteem.

It is probably not within the scope of your capability to prescribe medication for yourself and any such practice is very risky anyway. Often a small dose of medication may relieve your inner tension enough to be able to control the anxiety to allow you to think more about what is happening to you before you take any action. If the anxiety is so overwhelming that you are unable to think "through it" or in spite of it, then some emotional support may be helpful. However, from whomever you get that emotional support, that person cannot supply you with the neurophysiological means to overcome the anxiety. You have to do it, with or without the medication. The helper can only "hold your hand" for emotional support. He cannot do it for you. Trying to give you a reason why such an experience occurred, or blaming it on some memory or significant person in the past does nothing but postpone your confrontation with yourself to make your own change. Blaming it on the past is no excuse. You are responsible now for the manner in which you respond now.

To become independent you must feel that you <u>are</u> independent and capable of controlling your own affairs. You have to do your own swimming - or you sink into what you were previously. Independence in your neurophysiological system of living means swim or sink. Events occur in your life over which you have no control. However, you do have some control of the method and extent which you can exert in how you react to the uncontrollable event.

Because of the revolution in advancement of technology in examining the brain, as well as the entire body, some authors are proposing that the old specialty terms "neurology" and "psychiatry" as well as "neuropsychiatry" be abandoned in favor of a new term "neuropathiatry". Such a specialty would include all those physicians now certified in neurology or psychiatry. It would exclude neurosurgery because it would not include surgery of the brain. If such a suggestion were to be taken seriously it will be several years before we note any changes from our current terminology, and you can be sure, not without a considerable storm within both current professions.

Peschel, Enid, & Peschel, Richard E.
<u>Neuropathiatry: New Language Necessitated by the Neuroscience Revolution</u>
Perspectives in Biol & Med 38:183:(2) Winter 1995

CHAPTER 13

The only personality you have to work with when you decide you want to work out some of your problems is the personality with which you developed those tensions and anxieties in the first place and with which you have lived all your years. The chances of your getting over your tensions and anxieties in a hurry are very small.

You have to remember, it is the therapist's job to tell you what you do not want to hear. As a matter of fact, it is his job to tell you all those things you have tried not to listen to yourself, all the years you have been developing the kind of personality and the person you are. So, you are starting out to improve an imperfect person, having only that imperfect person with which to make the improvement.

To look at it another way, what ever system of adjustment you have made, not only protected you from some of those unpleasant sensations, feelings, and knowledge about yourself, but also, it was your attempt to express the dissatisfaction which you felt. It was your attempt to express those feelings even though the expression of those feelings was also imperfect.

So, how long it will take you to get yourself straightened out and get more satisfactions out of the system of expression which you developed no one can guess. As an improvement you will also want to feel more congenial and easy about yourself with what new adjustments you will have made. How quickly you can drop the old masks of deception and at the same time allow yourself to be more open and direct in the expression and satisfaction of your feelings will determine how long it will take you to change.

After all, what we try to do in developing our personality is express ourselves and prevent ourselves from being unacceptable at the same time. Most of us have a feeling if everybody knows what we are really like as a person, they may not like us and we want to be liked.

The probabilities are if we were more emotionally open and less frightened of what other people might think. we would be liked more quickly and more effectively, but that is not always true.

Some of us feel we are so angry and hostile inside we drive everybody away from us when they find out what we are like as people. Therefore, we try to disguise ourselves but in so doing we cannot avoid disguising ourselves to ourselves and that is what creates the problem.

Unless I can be honest with myself about what I am feeling, I have less chance of controlling my feelings and letting them be expressed in a more acceptable manner at the same time being able to get some satisfaction out of that expression. If I go to a therapist what I have to do is learn how to use that therapist to practice being able to be more direct and honest with myself in my expression, so I can feel more comfortable with that therapist and feel that the therapist will accept me anyway, in spite of my short comings.

I also have to have some feeling I am not going to destroy the therapist in my expression of anger. Nor am I going to destroy myself in the process and that may take a bit of doing.

It is a rare person indeed, who is aware of what I just said. All of the adjustments we learned to make as we were forming our personality and with which we have lived for however long we have lived, are out of our awareness. They are "unconscious", but we use them more effectively than if we were aware of what we are doing. The reactions by which we adjust are so rapid that we don't know we are reacting. They are "automatic" and it is that automatism we must face to be able to change.

That is what is difficult for us to accept when the therapist tells us how we are reacting and what he sees us expressing. We don't believe what the therapist says and we may become angry or frustrated with the therapist because the therapist is telling us something which we don't want to hear. That's the therapist's job, to tell us what we have spent our lives trying not to hear about ourselves.

The only measure of duration which the therapist controls is the predetermined issue of the length of each interview. In all other respects you, the supplicant, has total control over the contacts. It is true the so called therapist will set up a schedule to meet his needs, so far as duration of each interview is concerned, and may make recommendations regarding frequency. How many interviews will be involved over the numbers of weeks or months which will be needed will be totally under your control. There may be some exceptions in the event that a medication is used to try to shorten the total number of contacts with the therapist, then the medication will have a distinct effect. These days the managed care companies control how much they will pay and that can be a factor in the duration of your contact with the therapist., You always have the option of paying for the interviews yourself.

In recent years, medication has made a great improvement over what used to occur, because the medication helps to relieve your tension much more frequently and quickly than just interviewing alone will do. However, medication is a double edged sword, in that its prescription may require some weeks or months to adjust appropriately for you.

There is no way to plan the content of any particular interview; there is no way to plan the content of a series of interviews in order to get at what's going on within you to relieve your tensions. The best that can occur is that the physician will make an estimate of what he feels the major physiological problem is within you and then he will prescribe what medication he feels is the most appropriate for your particular circumstances. The adjustment of medication for proper dosage and for duration of effect may require some juggling over many weeks time. If you become frustrated and impatient because you expect the medication to have a quick effect and that does not occur and you leave the therapy, then you may be doing yourself a disservice, rather than a help.

The therapist and you have to work together in order to arrive at a dosage of medication in which the side effects are at a minimum and the desired therapeutic effect is at a optimum. The adjustment of dosage of medication may require several months of selecting and trying different dosages of perhaps the same medicine before a more or less ideal dosage schedule is arrived at to your satisfaction.

When it comes to interviewing, since there is no way to plan which content of what interview may be effective, you may always feel uncomfortable, because what you would like to do is to get it over with and to be changed in some manner or another as quickly as possible.

Fortunately, the therapist has no capacity to change you. The therapist can only work with you so that you can investigate yourself.

In terms of numbers of interviews, each of which may make very small progress, at a very irregular rate, there is no way to predict the number of interviews required to recognize any perceptible change in yourself. The rate of progress is a function of you, not of the interviewer. You always have control of what happens during the interview and at any time you may stop or alter the interview at your will.

We must remember that the fundamental effective contact in the interviews is the emotional exchange between the therapist and you, or that you are using the therapist to investigate yourself in so far as being able to express your emotions and finding a trust in the therapist to allow you to be dependent or vulnerable as well as verbally assertive depending on the circumstances in what is going on in you at that particular point in time.

The therapist has no way of stimulating the real feeling that must be expressed in the course of the treatment.

What the medication does in these circumstances is to attenuate the strength of your feelings to a point where they are much more manageable and perhaps more direct and balanced in the expression of affection, of anger, of hostility, or what ever is the predominate feeling at the time. Unfortunately, one of the side effects of many of the antianxiety medications which are available today is the impediment of memory which can occur.

Such diminution of memory is not constructive, but at the same time it can be utilized constructively because it does help you to react more realistically in the immediate circumstances of the interview itself.

There is no quick reliable solution. Nor can there be a planned progress of the conduct of the interviews in order for them to be most effective. It must be that they just proceed along their own lines, going from one topic to another, depending on what the mood is between the two participants at any particular time.

Of course there is always one question which is "when do you know when to stop, when is the treatment complete"? The treatment is complete when you or the therapist feels the treatment is complete. Unfortunately, there are some circumstances in which the therapist fails to retain a certain emotional distance by allowing you to become so dependent on him that you may feel there may be no time when you will be able to act independently. Then you may get a feeling of inability to take responsibility for yourself. When such dependency happens one set of circumstances of maladjustment have been substituted for the original set of maladjustments.

One of the therapist's jobs is to assist you in breaking the contacts and becoming independent. As there comes a time in all of our lives when we must become independent of our parents in order to live our own lives, so it is in treatment. You must become independent of the therapist to live your own life and to find out whether or not the therapy itself has been of any use in making that independent adjustment.

Factually, just because the interviews stop in frequency and duration does not mean that the therapy itself has come to an end. What it does mean is that you should carry away with you the kernel of the new adjustment and should test those new adjustments against your lifestyle and your life's events as they come and go. It may take several months and even several years before the full effect of the therapy can be realized even though direct contact with the therapist has ended. When a break comes in a series of contacts with the therapist, that is a period when you must begin to make use of and try to apply what you have learned about yourself in real life situations, rather than just in the office during the interviews. You are ready to get out on your own. Such learning about yourself usually takes some time and it may take several years after the therapy has "come to an end" before you really begin to function at a level which is most efficient for you at a new level of adjustment.

In a sense, the therapy never comes to an end. Hopefully, if the therapy in the office is successful, you will spend the rest of your natural life with a kind of a "split personality", and in which some part of you will remain aloof and be constantly trying to assess what the effects of your behavior is on the people around you and hopefully, simultaneously, be able to make adjustments to the constant evaluation which you are making of yourself. At the same time you will be able to relax, enjoy your feelings and be free of major anxiety.

We should never be free of all anxiety. Anxiety is a protective device for every living being. Without it we are totally vulnerable to the vicissitudes of the world, and those who would literally prey on us. Benjamin Franklin is credited with saying "the price of liberty is eternal vigilance". Such eternal vigilance is anxiety and in their own way plants exhibit a similar type of vigilance as they lean toward sunlight to capture the sun's rays for survival.

It is not unusual that after a period of time, you will show up in the therapist's office, if he is still available, and attack some new problem or a new period of adjustment with confidence, because you know the therapist will not try to impose his standards on you, but that the therapist will assist you in finding your own level, at a higher level of emotional maturity, that you may return with confidence to the real world.

When such relapses occur, you usually do not expect the therapist to provide any kind of answer. From the previous learning experience in therapy, you expect the therapist to assist you in working out your own problems and the relationship is a much more realistic and fruitful one. Usually a few interviews at that level are sufficient to allow you to make that adjustment to the new situation and then proceed with your life better than it possibly could have, had you not returned to the therapist. You may not need to go back to the therapist, if your therapy had been completely successful some part of your thinking apparatus will be set into activity and you may well be able to reassess yourself, to be more honest with yourself and arrive at a better reassessment than when you became aware of your more than necessary discomfort.

No person's life goes completely smoothly. Each of us, at different times in our lives, has crises which we meet. Regardless whether they are thrust upon us, or we make them for ourselves it is up to us to resolve them and to proceed with our life as best we can and live or die with the consequences. We are constantly making decisions of one kind or another throughout the course of life and such decisions are necessary and unavoidable.

The therapy only becomes interminable when the therapist fails to assist you in assuming the responsibility for yourself and if the therapist encourages you to become dependent upon him to make those decisions, then he is only thinking of himself and his future income and his future personal satisfaction.

If the therapist gets some vicarious or indirect pleasure out of having a number of people dependent on him, the therapist is doing you a considerable disservice and the therapy truly does become interminable until such time when you rebel against your own inner dependency and with a great deal of turmoil, leave the therapy often without the consent of the therapist or even without his blessing. Freud and his follower's recognized this potential and recognized that the therapy had failed when it becomes interminable. In the psychoanalytic system of thinking there is no recognition that the therapist has failed the patient. From the analytic point of view, you had failed yourself. In my view, what I think of as intermittent therapy, is the successful conclusion of your treatment at a point in time at which you may intermittently, at unpredictable intervals, need to reassess yourself in terms of the life you have at that particular time which has created new tensions or anxieties.

If the therapy has been successful you would be able to do that on your own, continue to make decisions, take off in different directions if necessary, and make adjustments as life proceeds. Occasionally, this intermittency does require you to return to the therapist for a kind of a reassessment, with the therapist's assistance, in making which ever new adjustment you may need to make. I do not consider a need to reassess yourself a failure of the therapy or your failure. When the therapy does finally come to an end, you will be able to relinquish the need to return to the therapist for that kind of reassurance or that kind of a reassessment. What actually happens is that you find sources in life other than the therapist which you use and with which, without returning to the therapist, make your decisions and continue with your life as best you can with the satisfaction which you are trying to find.

There are a group of therapists who now advocate what they call SST (Single Session Therapy).The entire system of therapy is based on one session of psychotherapy, and only one. They claim that that is enough to get their "clients" out of their ruts and into a more productive life. They say that more than one session is taking advantage of the client. They do not eliminate the possibility that at some time in the future there may be a need for you to return for another single session. Many people who have tried the system are available to testify that they have gone on living for several years with the changes they were able to make during that single session. Many claim they were cured. But with all such claims one must ask the people with whom they live whether a single session was sufficient to make as many changes in them as they seem to feel they made. Frequently, the people with whom they live may not give whole hearted support to the client's assertion that they were cured by that single session. There may very well be a difference of opinion on that appraisal. It is possible but less frequent than the authors of the system proclaim.

Through out your contacts with the therapist most of the interviews may seem dull and boring and you may well wonder what is happening, if anything. Such frustration with the process is not at all unusual.

However, every now and then an interview will come along during which you may see some of the same content of your thought in a different meaning, as though a light had come on where only darkness prevailed before. It may come as a surprise to you that a different meaning to the same thought had happened. Such events in changes of meaning are called "insight". They are not only new thoughts. They may also reflect a new emotional meaning to you. The new emotional meaning may leave you with the feeling that you had been a fool, or worse, for never having recognized the new meaning previously. Such feelings of recrimination are frequent, but also short lived. You may feel that a whole new world has opened up to you as the implications of the new meaning spread to other aspects of your life and you begin to recognize how you had arranged your life around the old system and now that you have seen the new the old meaning is lost.

These bits and pieces of changes from new "insight" are what make up the therapy. They can not be planned nor predicted. They are the stepping stones toward rearranging your life because prior to the time of the expression of new understanding you were spending much emotional energy in preventing such recognition from entering consciousness. Now, you have that suppressive energy available for more constructive use. You don't need it anymore for suppression.

Not all systems of conduct of therapy lead to such sharp recognition of insight. But therapy is based on such changes however insidious they occur. Without them there is no therapy because you do not change otherwise. Whether such pieces occur in or out of formal treatment is not the least bit important. Ideally the therapist is trying to equip you to conduct your own such therapy without anyone else being present.

When you have arrived at this stage you have become emotionally mature and independent. It requires a constant need and expression of energy to maintain that status. Keep swimming.

CHAPTER 14

Now comes the time to think about who is going to be able to afford all this treatment and new found independence.

It used to be that it was a very simple and straight forward proposition - that the person who needed the help went in to see the physician and the physician set his fees for that particular person's income as well as he could, or what he thought his services were worth in a particular economy. He told the patient what it would cost per treatment hour and they agreed in a verbal contract to see one another. At the end of each month the physician presented the patient with the bill and it was the patient's obligation to pay the bill before the tenth of the following month or the contract would come to an end.

Freud established that system of monthly payments and it had become universal for psychiatrists since about 1910. Further, it was implicit in the verbal agreement that the patient had contracted for the physician's time. The physician was obligated to appear on time, and the patient paid for the time whether he was able to meet the appointment or not. If he notified the physician at least 24 hours in advance and thereby released that block of time for the physician to use some other way he was released from payment. If the physician was late by ten or more minutes the patient was not obligated to pay. If the patient left the appointment early, at his own initiative, he was obligated to pay for the entire appointment time. Should the physician be ten or more minutes late and an agreement made that the physician would compensate the patient for an equal amount of time at another time, the payment for the appointment was due. There had to be mutual verbal agreement arrived at the first interview.

The system has changed. People do not seem to feel responsible for their contracts with the physician, in so far as paying the physician is concerned.

Most patients feel that it is the insurance company's responsibility to pay the physician and it is the physician's problem to collect from the insurance company. It is very difficult for patients to learn that they are responsible for themselves, which includes being responsible for paying the bill.

It is especially true that people who are older feel that it is now the government's responsibility to pay the bill; that they themselves have no financial responsibility because of their age and the government's promise to pay through Medicare and Medicaid. With Medicare and Medicaid as the pattern, the "third party payers" have also changed their patterns of payment for practically all ages of people seeking medical and psychiatric help. Our federal government has taught the public that it is no longer responsible to care for itself; at least all those folks on Medicare and Medicaid.

Furthermore, the Federal Government has now mandated, by regulation and law, that the physician is responsible to submit the request for payment for the patient, and the patient is not responsible even for that. The Government has decreased the independence of the patient by so ordering.

Over the past several decades this general condition has come about because the federal government has said to the people that you are not responsible for yourselves. We will take care of you and such programs as Medicare and Medicaid, which presumably is to take care of those people who are "unable to care for themselves".

The government has now made promises to the people that it, the government, will now pay the bill and has created a national debt which is so substantial that it is choking the total national economy and bringing the country to insolvency. It is by this means the congress has been reelected 98% of the time and in the process has killed incentive for individuals to feel they are responsible for themselves and their lives whether they like it or not. Taxes have also risen, but the public cannot afford to pay all the tax money needed to pay the deficit as created by expenditures.

Now we have reached the stage where the congress is in a dilemma because it is not able to take a realistic look at what are euphemistically called "entitlement programs".

These entitlement programs are nothing but the federal deficit which the congress has created over the past 60 years to lead people down a primrose path, telling you that you are not responsible for yourselves. We, your elected representatives to the congress, are responsible for you and we will tax you in accordance with how much we feel you should be taxed in order to foot the bills which we appropriate. Those appropriations are all free, except to you as a tax payer and a working person. You have to foot the bills for all such appropriations by paying more taxes.

It is like going into a restaurant together, you and your members of congress, senators and representatives, at which time they say we will evenly split the papers brought to the table. I will take the menu and you the bill.

This is what has happened in psychiatry and generally, in all of medicine. You, as a patient, seem to feel you are not responsible for the debt you create when you go to see the psychiatrist. You are not responsible for yourself or your own welfare and you have been told so frequently even by third party insurance carriers, as well as by the federal government itself, that you are not a financially responsible individual. The only people who pay the taxes are those people who try to take care of themselves by earning their living outside the largesse of the federal government. The remainder of the people feel the federal government owes them their living from the taxes collected and the appropriations which are not funded by taxes, but are debts.

Also included in that list of people and organizations who told you that you are not responsible for yourself, are the unions. The unions have told the various employers that if you, the employer, don't give us, the employees, "free" medical insurance we, the union, will go on strike and cause the company to go defunct. The congress has supported this "free "medical care by eliminating the medical insurance programs paid by the company from employee's income taxes, thus making them "free" of income tax liability.

The company managers have agreed with what is euphemistically called "negotiated" medical payments and now those medical payments through the insurance carriers, and the unions, have gotten so high that, in some cases, it costs more for medical insurance premiums than it does to build an automobile or what ever else is being built.

The so called "fringe benefits" may be more expensive than the item itself. This has succeeded in allowing you to get yourself off the hook and say someone else is responsible. Furthermore, the payments which your medical insurers contribute to your medical costs are not taxable. One of the results is that you seek medical care more often than you would otherwise and thus medical costs are increased by more frequent, and sometimes unnecessary, medical care. You have also abdicated the responsibility to give simple medical care to yourself and your family, and have instead just said "go to the Doctor. It's all free". It is free at the price of your independence.

Likewise, Medicare and Medicaid have expanded to include many other programs to supply "free" income derived from debt dollars. Almost anyone who can stagger into a physician's office and say that "I am not able to work anymore and being not able to work, it is the government's responsibility to take care of me. I should have SSI or disability government payments".

The facts are that a significant portion of individuals who are on Medicare and Medicaid are quite capable of working and have no physical disability. A mental disability may become a disability only because one believes that one is not able to work, rather than be unable to work although there are many mentally disabled who, truly, are unable to work. A large number of people who are mentally ill are quite capable of holding down some kinds of jobs, but so long as the SSI pays them more than they could earn in the open job market they are not about to take a cut in income to go to work.

Now, some government agencies buy advertisements to inform the public that it is "entitled" to debt dollars although it isn't stated that way in the ads. All of these attitudes in persuading you that you are not able to work or you are not capable of working has led you to believe that you are not. Because if you believe you are unable to work you will be unable to work.

There are many people who are truly unable to work at the same types of jobs at which they were injured and they often have a hard time retraining themselves for new kinds of work, or finding the financial support they need while they are trying to retrain themselves. There are various types of retraining programs to fill this gap. Many such "rehabilitation" programs do include money for living expenses in addition to paying tuition for retraining.

Meanwhile, the government and the third party payers are saying that it is the physician's problem that medical care costs so much and taxes and premiums are so high and you are not able any longer to go and see a physician because he charges too much. To cure this problem of cost of physicians services, the government and third party payers have set fee schedules and the government has made it a criminal act, in some cases, for a physician to charge a patient any fee above that which the government approves. Nor can the physician refuse to accept such government fee schedules, or any fee from the government and make his contract for pay with the patient as an independent, responsible, person.

The other problem, in so far as mental health is concerned, is that psychologists, social workers, ministers and anybody who can write his own name legibly or illegibly for that matter, can hang out a shingle saying I am a "psychotherapist". Psychotherapy in and of itself does not include any kind of medical care but I, a "Mental Health Professional", do the same things the psychiatrist does and under these circumstances I, the "Mental Health Professional", should be paid the same fees that the psychiatrist receives. Some courts have accepted the testimony of non physicians as equal in expertise as that of physicians. With this attitude, which is so rampant around the United States, not only the physician, psychiatrist, needs to be paid out of what are called medical care costs but a lot of other people who have no relationship to medical care as far as their education and responsibility are concerned.

One of the events that may come about when you go to see such a "Mental Health Professional" and you get into emotional trouble in the course of the psychotherapy or you begin to talk about suicide or you talk about or actually do hurt someone, then that so called "mental health professional", mental health expert, licensed marriage counselor, licensed professional counselor or psychologist tells you to go to a doctor. By a doctor they do not mean a Doctor of Theology; they don't mean a Doctor of Psychology; they mean a physician, a psychiatrist.

At that point in time, the psychiatrist or other physician is saddled with the responsibility of getting you out of the problem that you have dug yourself into because you did not except the responsibility for yourself and feel you cannot do so in relation to a psychiatrist. The emotional situation for you is worse than when you began.

Under these circumstances, what has happened is that, you have lost your freedom. You are no longer the same free, independent, self sufficient individual who as a personality started this country looking for a better place to live for himself and his family. Independence means swim or sink. You have been seduced into sinking by the promise of an easier life based on someone else's effort.

What you have become, of course, is a puppet. You have allowed yourself to be seduced into the feeling that you are no longer responsible for your own welfare but that you want that welfare provided for you at no financial or emotional cost to yourself. No cost in labor, no cost in time. What you would like to do, of course, is live the same way you fantasize everybody else lives, the 60' yacht, enough land or lot to meet your wishes, a fancy house, and all the services you desire with little or no effort on your part. All of these "good things of life" with as little effort as possible.

You have traded your independence for "security" which is not that secure. This also means that if you get physically sick then someone else is responsible for taking care of you and it is not your responsibility to care for yourself.

The essence is that you have lost your freedom. You have given it away to be dependent on someone else to give you your freedom. No one else can give you freedom. No one can "give" you psychotherapy or medical care. You can't buy psychotherapy. All you can buy is an opportunity to straighten yourself out and that means effort on your part in earning the money or having it come from somewhere, such as your own effort and work to create personal investments and seeing to it that those investments work for you. You must manage the investments which do bring money in to you that you may pay those bills out of your own pocket from your own earnings.

Of course, it is extremely difficult for you to do this because all these years taxes have increased insurmountably to such a point where now a significant part of your working year is devoted to paying taxes and paying the interest on the moneys which the government has borrowed. All those items and services which you feel you are due, the yacht, new appliances, new cars, a house in which you would like to live, federal "grants", loans, disability payments to all those people who are not disabled, and large federal pensions to the congressmen and federal employees who appropriated the indebtedness and were paid by it, you bought, with interest. You seem to feel that you are not responsible for paying the interest or the debt any more. You are not responsible for actually generating the income to take care of yourself.

Very few people feel that they are responsible for themselves and have to make the adjustment necessary to do their own living. They want someone else to do the paying for them, but they want to get all the pleasure out of it, without expending the effort.

Retailers have a phrase "The customer is always right". Well, that is excellent. You are the customer but you are also the retailer. Unless you retail your wares, the emotional, physical and mental assets you have, you are not likely to have the income to satisfy the customer.

In order to get the most out of your assets, whatever they are, it is necessary for you to make a personal examination to identify your needs, capabilities and assets and to also identify your marketing techniques so that you can get the most out of your assets as far as your emotional income is concerned.

It is not constructive to believe that the federal government owes you your medical care or that the state or federal government owes you an income and it is all their fault because the check is late this month. It is not their fault. It is your fault because you allow them the privilege of creating your check with borrowed money.

Employers can't pay you for spending time in their factory. What they pay you for is the work you do while you are there. Unless the work you do while you are there is worth paying for, there is no good reason for them to pay for it.

To be independent and free you must take the risks to manage yourself. The world economy is such that unless we are productive for the amount of time we spend trying to produce something or perform some service, or create some item or service which others desire and are willing to buy, we cannot compete with other people who live in other advanced industrial nations.

Each day you go to work you do not work for your own income until approximately 10:00 am if you work on a 7:00 am to 3:30 PM schedule (an 8 hour day). It takes 3 1/2 hours of each 8 hour work day to pay your taxes.

It is also true that in some nations medical care of any kind, including absolute necessities, is not available to buy. It is because of the competition amongst physicians that the medical care that is available is available even though the cost appears to be high. The quality of the care you are receiving is the best that people have ever received in the history of man. Now, and for several years, the costs of medical care are escalating far faster than any other segment of the economy and constitute a substantial portion of the entire federal budget. Yet, not all the increased costs for medical care are directed to paying for medical care. Recently the individual charged by Federal Government with the responsibility to dispense national funds for Medicare and Medicaid revealed that that agency does not know what the administrative costs are to supervise the entire funds.

It is estimated that other systems for the delivery and payment of medical are less expensive per person than ours. Yet, in none of those systems is the patient able to freely select the physician of his choice and obtain whatever care he needs, particularly hospital care, when he needs it. He must wait in line for diagnostic tests and for treatment. Psychiatric care is greatly limited under those plans and many people pay for private psychiatric care rather than subject themselves to the delays and unknown quality of the care which is furnished by the government.

Nature does not permit survival in a negative balance. Every plant and animal which survives must live in a neutral or positive balance or death is inevitable. Healing cannot occur in a negative balance. Yet, people seem to feel that it is not necessary for them to live on what income they have. They seem to believe that they can go into debt, pay the price of the interest on the borrowed money, live and "get ahead".

I believe that people, governments, societies all must live on what they take in. If the costs of what they take in are too high they will have a negative balance and will not survive. People who make poor adjustments expend too much of their emotional energy trying to live from day to day and unless they live free of emotional debt they can not compete. They perish. They sink.

When the payments are too high there is not sufficient left over on which to survive, so economy in the expenditure of our emotional assets is necessary. We must also have some pleasure as a part of survival and pleasure time and quality is the reward for efficient living. When our emotional costs demand more than we are able to generate in emotional income, we are in real trouble and then is the time to reexamine how we are generating the income and we are spending the wages. Nothing comes without the expenditure of effort, and the price is high. Fortunately, for some people they are able to be naturally more efficient than others and do not apparently need to work so hard at survival. But each pays in his own way. Nothing is for free. Independence means swim or sink.

Friedman, Milton
<u>Gammon's Law Points to Health Care Solutions</u>
Wall Street Journal, Vol:LXXXVIII #95 Tuesday Nov. 12 1991

CHAPTER 15

Many times over the years people have asked, "What do I do if I meet you socially ?".

The answer is: be yourself. Never mind that you are a patient; never mind that you are coming in for treatment; never mind that you are feeling particularly close or distant depending on what the circumstances are at the time. Forget all that. After all, we are just people. You are people. I am people. There is absolutely no reason you should feel particularly uncomfortable, even though I know you do, when we happen to meet in public.

I'm sure whenever we happen to meet in public, you begin to feel everybody in the room knows "I am going to see a psychiatrist, and this particular psychiatrist", or "I had seen this psychiatrist". That they know is simply not true.

It is not true because there is no way that anybody else can know unless you tell them. You can tell them in various and different ways. You can tell them by word of mouth. You can say "I'm going to see this man as a patient", or you can tell them by your embarrassment and behavior and the manner in which you relate while we are in that social situation, but it doesn't make any difference how you tell. You can tell them by your facial expressions; by changes in your usual motions when you are talking about something else; by shuffling your feet or by waving your arms, by any motion which you alter from your usual motions in talking. Catches in your voice, changes in tone, hesitations, too rapid or too slow speech may let the cat out of the bag.

If you feel at ease you won't let anyone else know that you are seeing me or had seen me professionally.

I feel it is nobody else's business. I am not going to tell them and I will relate to you as a person, not from what I know in the office, but just from whatever is going on at that particular point in time and unless something very unusual comes up, no one around us will know you have been coming to talk to me. I think any other psychiatrist you go to that you meet in a social situation will feel essentially the same way. Unless you become so embarrassed you give yourself away, no one else will realize that you have become or were a patient.

There is only one way possible for someone to realize that you are a patient and that is if you have identified with me; adapted some of my mannerism's; adapted some of my tone's of voice, some of my speech habits, some of my style of dressing, some of the other quirks of my personality and you have not realized that you have adopted. Someone else might look at the two of us and feel that in effect, you are copying me and they would also recognize you do not know you are copying me, but they would know for sure you are now, or were, a patient of mine.

This copying process and state is called identification. I can remember one time seeing a man on the street whom I knew as a friend. He was not a patient of mine, but he was a patient of a friend of mine, another psychiatrist. I saw him walking down the street and I knew for certain that he had become a patient of this friend of mine, because of the manner in which he walked. He had copied the particular swing of his psychiatrist's walk. Whenever he walked, he walked with exactly the same kind of mannerisms, the swing in which he moved his arms and his body in the process of walking. The friend of mine, himself, was completely unaware of it and I did not mention it to him. To have mentioned it would have only created more problems than it would have solved.

You may also wonder if somebody asks point blank, whether or not you have been coming to see me or some other psychiatrist, then what do you do? You do what you want to do. If you want them to know, you tell them. I feel it is nothing to be ashamed of, even though I know that going to see a psychiatrist is now far more acceptable than it used to be. There is still a tremendous social stigma in some people's thinking about going to see a psychiatrist. Most people are more fearful of losing their minds than they are of being mortally ill.

Frequently, people will feel that if they have to go to see a psychiatrist, that means that they are totally crazy and no one will want to have anything to do with them and will avoid them at all costs. It is because they are more fearful of losing their mind and being unacceptable to the world, than they are of having a physical disease which might cause them to die. In the event that you have these feelings, that you would rather be dead than to go to see a psychiatrist, the likelihood of a psychiatrist being able to help you is considerably reduced. In the event you do overpower your fear of going and try to help yourself the likelihood of you're helping yourself is greatly enhanced. You have made the biggest step toward helping yourself, getting help. Unless you can look at yourself somewhat objectively and feel it is a necessary step for you to take toward emotional maturity in going through life, the chance of your being helped by psychiatry is relatively small.

The psychiatrist is simply another person and it makes no difference whether you meet him in the office, in a hall, in a public building, at a party, wherever it is that you meet him, he is simply another person and you are a person in your own right and are subjected to the same kinds of feelings the psychiatrist is, or anybody else. There is no reason for you to feel embarrassment because you happen to inadvertently run into him some place.

I know that what I am writing now will not influence you to any significant degree, and probably you will feel embarrassed. I assure you that is your own appraisal of what is happening to you and your own dislike of what's happening to you; dislike of the fact that you need to go to see someone at all or at any particular point in your life has as much if not more effect on you than what I am writing here.

Different techniques of managing yourself have been suggested to avoid the feeling of embarrassment. It makes no difference how you do it. The key is your own self confidence. When you can feel that you are the equal of anyone else, including the psychiatrist, then you will not be embarrassed. Of course, what took you to the psychiatrist in the first place was the lack of confidence in yourself. Straighten your tie, smooth your dress, pat your hair in place, throw back your shoulders, whatever you do to give yourself the confidence to meet him face on and do it.

How you came to lack self confidence is what most of the theories of psychiatry are all about. And they are that, theories.

How you came to lack confidence in yourself is dependent on your life's story and how you managed yourself in the tests of life through which everyone passes, or the tests of life through which you passed and are special to your life and which everyone manages differently. So, it might be said that your feeling of embarrassment in being in a social situation with your psychiatrist is no different from any other event in your life and you managed it by feeling embarrassed. Managing your feelings in a social situation will help you gain self confidence. You are the equal of anybody else. What you are doing is practicing feeling the equal of anyone else. That practice also gradually gets easier as the number of times you do it increase. You will fall into the habit of not feeling embarrassed. You will feel more comfortable and soon you will not have that feeling of anxiety which prevented you from seeing him in public when you avoided going places where he might be. You might come to enjoy seeing him. Feeling embarrassed is just another symptom. It represents an attempt on your part to hide your feelings and to express them at the same time. It is the expression of what Helmut Kaiser called "duplicity", the universal symptom of neuroses. It is trying to hide your true feeling by disguising them in some way so that other people will not know. If you are afraid of being hostile to someone else you may try to hide that hostility, but hiding hostility can never be completely accomplished. Nor can ignoring it. So in trying to keep the seriousness of your hostility hidden you develop a symptom, become embarrassed, flush, faint, shake, stutter, tremble, or something else if that hostility is too strong or too near the surface that it threatens to burst out of you with angry language or very insulting remarks or something similar.

The basic feeling doesn't have to be hostility. You could come to admire him and not want anyone to recognize it. The same limits will apply. You will be able to partially hide your feelings and partially express them simultaneously. If anyone notices it will be because you have given yourself away in your expression.

The worst scenario will be that the other guests might be amused at your plight. Otherwise, it won't bother them. If they feel somewhat close to you they might make a remark or two to kid you about the situation. Such social interplay is most often in the spirit of sharing not of chiding. It is as though they are saying "I know what you are feeling, I've been in that situation too". Or "I am glad it is happening to you and not to me". They often feel less stilted toward you and you will feel the increased warmth and camaraderie. Although at the time you may feel like crawling under the carpet.

Kaiser, Helmut Effective Psychotherapy
The Contribution of Helmut Kaiser
Ed: Louis B. Fierman M.D.
The Free Press, New York, 1965
Collier-Macmillan, Limited.   London

CHAPTER 16

Man's eternal problem, in a sense damnation, is the fact that each generation must learn from birth and go through the developmental process of intellectual growth and emotional adjustment in the process of getting to be adult, until death, just as does every living creature of whatever species. Combined with the burden of the increasing complexity of what goes on, each generation is saddled with the inexorable developmental cycle which zoologists have recognized for many years as existing developmentally and embryologically. "Ontogeny recapitulates Phylogeny".(The embryological development of the individual goes through all the phases of the evolutionary development of all the phyla which preceded it.)

That being the case there is no possibility, at least as we know now, of producing an organizational base for birth and development which would allow man to proceed from where the last generation left off as a foundation for the level at which the new generation begins. Each mammalian generation proceeds from a biological beginning in utero and repeats the entire developmental cycle beginning with a single cell organism. In utero, in the embryo, the individual develops through all the evolutionary stages until it reaches that stage of development for its species and then it emerges into the world to continue development into the adult of its species. So does mankind.

This is, in my feeling, one of the biggest detriments and at the same time the salvation of man. It is the cause of both growth and adaptability and also the extinction of species when a species fails to adapt to survive. Each generation must make infinitely small changes to adapt. Nature provides many variations in each generation and eventually the most adaptable are the only ones left. Mother nature's changes occur in the genes not in social adaptability. Which gene reflects the social adaptability is the one that survives.

The problems and speed with which development and alterations can occur in genes as well as in the social systems with conformity, as well as diversity, of individual personalities and complexities can be so rapid it may be utterly impossible for individuals to adapt to the world or the universe rapidly enough to ensure species or individual survival. Even now, our technological advances may have a very detrimental effect on adaptability except on a very few individuals. The majority of persons born today, have such a limited potential to grasp the complexities of the technological state in which we now exist that only a few are able to fully understand what is possible with our present knowledge.

Such a statement assumes that at present we are in command of the bulk of knowledge and assuredly we are not. We are progressing toward more capacity for knowledge and complexity of knowledge at a faster rate than has ever been achieved. It is said that our knowledge base now doubles every 3 years. Our knowledge base is only a minuscule fragment of what goes on to make the world work. As a wild guess, it seems to me that in the past 25 years, dated prior to 1990 and since, that 95% of man's knowledge has been discovered and it's impossible for any single individual to encompass even a significant fraction of the amount of knowledge that is available now.

Then, there is also the possibility of not being able to make the moral judgments and the philosophical applications of knowing which might be improvement in our lives or which could be detriment to our biological and social survival in the future.

If we ever forget that man is a biological entity arisen from some evolutionary or theological base, which argument and discussion I am not intending to get into now other than to partially present a portion of the biological entity, we shall be lost.

The fact that it takes two people, a male and a female, to conceive and the female to bear the burden of the gestation and delivery is daily evidence of our heritage. The period of gestation of nine months is determined by our biological heritage, but that, too, may not be forever for as we evolve it may be altered.

If man is ever able to substitute, I should say simply copy, the conditions of nurturing in the womb so that artificial gestation might occur outside the human body with a positive survival rate, the world will not be the same, nor will we. It is possible that should test tube pregnancy become routine, that mankind would stagnate at that point in evolution as biological evolution would be artificially selected by a few individuals who might very well decide amongst themselves, or in some cases alone, that a particular change in the genes of offspring might be an improvement. Unfortunately, by the time any one found out what the result of those changes might be, it may be too late.

Such arbitrary changes might not be an improvement but that fact might not be discovered for several generations after the fact.

I believe it is true that the universe will not be the same because we may be able to make better use of our capacities of intelligence than as of now. The technological advances of the 20th century have been so expansive compared with the technological advances which existed in all the previous time of mankind, that there is just no adequate comparison.

I limit this speculation to the 25 years just preceding 1990 for simplification. Fantasies of science fiction writers on paper have predicted the kinds of advances which mankind can make beyond the limit of our capability at the time of prediction. Socrates fantasized a relatively complete system and description of the atomic theory but had not the technical means to demonstrate the composition of matter. (Van Melsen) Now it is done "everyday".

Such fantasies are science fiction only because at the time they are published they have reached a state of complexity in prediction of which a large percentage of the population is not capable of initiating on it's own. The fantasies which some people are able to mentally conceive as innovations have no real bearing on what their personal capabilities are except that they have somehow found a way by which they can put "known" facts together mentally and come up with conclusions which other people can not. Whether such fantasies are predictions or whether they are simply new solutions to the same old problems, or new problems, is one of the fundamental philosophical questions which man will face when this kind of intelligence is dominant. At that time man may lose his humanness, because without those emotional charges which accompany his intelligence to make the best use of his intelligence to progress, he will be lost in a universe of pure reason and be something less than human.

Most emotional charges are triggered as a result of hormonal functions as well as neuronal functions. When hormonal functions no longer determine man's destiny, his individual life loses a great deal of the emotional warmth, interchange, and communication on which his biological development has been based for many years, particularly in interrelationship, one to the other.

Under such circumstances, the loss of emotional warmth and feelings, and hatreds, may cause life to become dull, gray, neutral and impersonal.

With that background man's identity as an individual will be lost. It will become a mechanical existence based on intellectual functions which man has not created by any means, but has expanded by the addition of a tremendous amount of "Knowledge" and what constitutes fact will have to be determined by intellectual description and not by any kind of emotion, opinion or indecision. There will be no room for doubt because everything will be picked out and selected and what the "Truth" is will be so well defined and so well specified that there will be no room for controversial presentations of tangential matter or inconclusive functions. No doubts about anything. What are "Facts" now will become myths in the future. Just as the "facts" of the past are now looked upon with humor and jocular tolerance, as myths.

All of the concepts, and feelings of psychiatric problems that have occurred will have automatically been eliminated because of the cold, ruthless, impenetrable indifference of intellectual fact. The lack of partiality, in all respects automatically, kills the life and the warmth and the emotional exchange which has to go on between people in order for them to be happy or to have any feelings of accomplishment. Such emotions as fear, anger and love will have been lost in the shuffle of pure intellectual impartiality.

The question arises then, should ultimate destiny depend on that kind of cold, ruthless impartiality, as to who will be making the decisions and as to which direction mankind will go?

It seems paradoxical that there can be a tremendous intellectual upheaval which could possibly be resolved by the total destruction of any rivalry if there is difficulty in arriving at a consensus as to planned destiny for the masses.

I can envision this as an autocracy, such as the feudal existence in the past, when the feudal governmental systems were united into monarchies, empires or kingdoms from which democracy has evolved presumably endowing the individual with the right to make his own decisions and exercise his own will. When intelligence becomes so universal that it will be equally divided, or at least each individual will have as much intelligence as every other individual, there can be tremendous upheaval. I feel it would be virtually impossible to totally eliminate affect or feelings, that go into making some decisions for any particular person or group of individuals of a few people who would subjugate all others and have the potential to destroy the world.

It would be a very poor world in which to live where there were no differences of opinion and pure intelligence could only lead to the small differences of opinion which would have been left from our biological heritage. Our biological heritage having been blown into oblivion, would be dominated by crass intelligence over the entire world. It would be an upheaval with the technological advantages or "The Technological Potentials" for destruction of the universe as well as of the world.

The utopia of Sir Francis Bacon is a fantasy in itself and many have speculated that Bacon wrote it as satire. The only possibility of salvaging man then would be to have some reproductive process loosed in the world, which would be exemplified by Jung's conceptualizations about the DNA and RNA data base being incorporated, at the time of conception, or before, into a system whereby the experiences of the individual as he goes through life would be integrated into the genetic structure and projected onto the new generation to give the new generation the higher intellectual and emotional level of integration where the old generation leaves off, or to eliminate any subsequent genetic variations.

How fast such a process could be incorporated into the conception and gestation of each individual, of course, is at this point unknown.

Such a system would leave the individual with virtually no sense of individual identity. Total intellectual functions would dominate. It would be an emotionally, extremely cold, unpleasant world, indeed, for those who had any emotion or feeling towards their fellow human beings.

Under those circumstances it might be possible, if the technological advances continued to accrue at the rate at which they have in these past 25 years, that the biological entity of conception within a living body would not be necessary, in that those functions could be carried out in a laboratory. If that were the case and we did reach that stage of development, then someone would have to make decisions about what type laboratory, and which genetic pool from which to select in order to newly develop and expand the base on which the future generations of mankind would be based, or to create a new, different genetic pool artificially. Stagnation could also set in by creating genes which could eliminate any changes in other genes.

There might be a kind of a philosophical and moral limitation as to the type of individual who would be developed, and of course the other possibilities would probably be automatically eliminated depending on the choice of the selector. Natural adaptation would be lost and mankind would be doomed because of a "natural" lack of capacity for adaptability.

When we think about these possible developments our individual, minor, day to day frustrations and limitations seem minuscule compared with the potential for "Success" and also for damage if such control were vested in a single being which could only be a "super" being.

As I have tried to discuss previously, such a super being would be in every individual who survived, or if bred out, totally lacking and the ultimate result would be ultimate destruction for all but one super being.

However, for that one it might no longer be necessary to have two people for procreation, or two biological entities for procreation, because the technological advances might have also reached a point where artificial DNA and RNA, as far as mankind is concerned, would be developed so that that, too, would be a clone of what the original biological entity of mankind started to be and where it came from. As the software writers for our relatively new computers are wont to say "garbage in, garbage out" and what constitutes garbage for one individual, or in this case one calculating machine and another calculating machine, could be completely and totally different. So, we are also, at this time of artificial intelligence getting to the point of being a totality and of itself, the destructive forces will be imbedded in the same trends and developments.

Now we have come full circle. We are now considering the good and the evil of the theologians and philosophers which have gone on for eons of mankind and it's questionable whether or not mankind could survive if there were the ultimate for total destruction as well as total survival. In a philosophical sense there is virtually no possibility of there being a totality of good in the world without there also being the totality for evil, because the predominance of good at that point would also be the evil of the destruction of everything else which would be in difference with it or in controversy with it.

Right at the moment we are back to our original conceptualization when I started writing this and that is that there is no compromise. Each and every step in "progress" has a price. In the very recent years (September 1992) a man was found frozen under the ice of a glacier in the Alps bordering Italy and Austria. He continues to be studied but it has been determined that he is approximately 5300 years old, between the ages of twenty-five and thirty-five years of age at the time of his death.

He is the oldest intact human found and his genetic structure, (DNA, Etc) is being studied by a motley group of anthropologists, world wide to determine how it differs from modern man, if it does. If it does not differ, it bodes a very slow process for the future changes in man.

This is particularly true when we are trying to investigate ourselves in order to "make better persons of ourselves". The ultimate dilemma is what is a better person, because in order to define what a better person is, it's also necessary for us to define what a worser person is.

Also, under these circumstances of this ultimate intellectual utopia, or infinity, there would be no beauty and no ugly; there would be no deformity and only all conformity; there would be no definitive better or worse; there would be no definable richer or poorer. There would be no definable smarter or dumber, because "mankind" would have reached a stage of ultimate uniformity and it would be impossible to discriminate these various dilemmas and various different categories.

Be thankful that you were nervous; be thankful that you were fearful; be thankful that you are frightened; be thankful that you have the capacity to love. Be thankful that you have the capacity to hate because that's what makes us human, without it we are nothing.

Which means that the power of positive thinking is the ultimate placebo and panacea and any system of thinking which encompasses only one aspect of these dilemmas and ignores the other aspect of dilemma dooms mankind. If there is a simple choice of one of two parts, then any aspect of such thinking automatically is a death trap at the same time it's a salvation.

George Bernard Shaw has been credited with saying the most difficult thing a man does in life is think and many people would rather die than think and they do.

Man is eternally destined to recapitulate the legend of the Phoenix and arise anew with each generation out of the ashes of the old. Unfortunately, man cannot arise from the peak or the epitome of the essence of completeness from the pinnacle of the previous generation but must in a sense return to ashes in order rise again.

In it's own way what I have just said also epitomizes the story of Christ and his crucifixion and rebirth, celebrating it as we do at Easter or in other religions the equivalent of death and rebirth. There would be no such things as introspection and self discipline and man would be inexorably bound to his destiny as dependent on the artificial intelligence and what it projects. Men who use their backs to earn their living put their backs at risk for injury and when injured it's usually their backs which receive the injury.

Men who use their minds to earn a living may also injure their minds. Unfortunately, the injured mind is not so readily discernible to the individual as the injured back. The injured mind very rarely puts out any specific pain which the individual recognizes but which those individuals around him may recognize long before he does. The injured mind also manifests it's injury into itself in the forms of delusions, hallucinations, deviations of thought processes, depression, anxieties, hyperactivity, mania and all these inner stirrings which the patient may feel and may experience but not recognize within himself as being the product of his own disturbance within his own mind. (Millar,T,P,)

Physical injuries are roughly divided into major injuries and minor injuries. The injuries of the mind may also be roughly divided into major injuries and minor injuries. Unfortunately, in both instances, the physical and the mental, there is a large gray area where it's often impossible to distinguish between the major and the minor injuries.

Furthermore, even a minor physical injury might extend itself into a major mind injury, because it's impossible to injure the body without having the mind, which is also a part of the body, affected.

On the other hand a major or minor mind injury might at the same time have a major impact on the body and create what appears to be a major or a minor physical injury with the primary source being the mind.

The distinctions between these two and the integration of the unity of the mind and the body is still being debated in medical, philosophical and particularly in psychiatric circles.

Without a doubt, professionals tend to separate the mind and the body. When they are "trained" they come out with a programmed notion that whatever it is in which they are trained is the only method, and they very rarely get enough education to be sufficiently expert in investigating both the mind and the body.

However expert they are in investigating the mind and the body, there remain limitations to both and no one is completely adequate in determining what injury is, in either the mind or the body, let alone together.

Millar, T.P. The Sterile Couch
Perspectives in Biol and Med 32,(2) 272-280 Winter 1989

Van Melsen, Andrew G.
From Atomos to Atom : The History of the Concept Atom
Harper & Brothers, N.Y. 1960: Torch Book 517

CHAPTER 17

The best way to achieve happiness in living is to think about yourself; think about what you would like to be, not what you are. It is necessary to be honest with yourself. You can start only with what you are. To start with dreaming what you would like to be or what kind of success you would like to have is impossible. To assess what your emotional assets are, what your physical assets are, what your social, financial and intellectual assets are, is only the beginning. Then, you can appraise what you are and how much you can or must change yourself to achieve the long term goals you set for yourself, to achieve what you would like to be. If you set no long term goals for yourself you are the equivalent of being weightless in space - no anchors.

Think about and define what you expect from life to be happy. Ideals alone do not lead directly to happiness. Happiness in fulfilling those dreams may be the very day to day, step by step, daily changes or fulfillments which when added together put you in and keep you in the state to which you aspire. Biological drives are the energy which drives us in the direction toward that goal of happiness.

In the privacy of your own mind, examine yourself honestly without embarrassment, including the most primitive of your life's functions eating, sleeping, urinating, defecating, sexual desires and satisfactions. Only you can scrutinize yourself to the extent which you need but if you are not honest with yourself you cannot begin on the path which will lead you to your goals. Independence means swim or sink.

As I indicated above these are some steps which I feel are needed if you are going to achieve something you would like to be.

One: You have to take an inventory.

Two: You have to make a statement of assets and liabilities, both mental and physical and be honest with yourself about whether or not you are positive or negative in both the physical as well as the mental aspects of you.

Three: Do the things your emotions tell you don't want to do but you know you must do. There are a lot of times in life when we have to do a lot of things we don't want to do but we know that it is absolutely necessary for us to do them in order to accomplish something or in order to do what we think is the right thing to do.

Four: Delineate in your own mind the types of affection that you enjoy or don't enjoy. That includes social interrelationships with the people you have contact with, the verbal interrelationships with the people you have contact with and to some extent the emotional and physical relationships you have. If you are not able to set yourself into two parts and experience what you are going through as well as think about it and recognize what it is, you are in for a great deal of trouble because you are set on a course of taking action without any real thought connected with it.

Five: You can not, you must not, give in to passion alone, either affection or anger. In this day and age we do not use the word passion in the manner which it originally was meant. Usually the word passion implies some kind of affection such as sexual passion but passion is just as appropriately applied to aggression or anger. If you allow yourself a limit of passion, angry, aggressive, depressive, euphoric as well as affectionate, then you are bound to have far more success in your life than you have had up until now. Passion implies an intensity of feeling, not the type of feeling. You must be able to express and control your passion and in order to do that. You must think before you act.

Six: Your self confidence comes from exploiting yourself in those parts of your personality which you like about yourself and if you can do that, then you will find confidence in yourself. On the other hand, just because you are mildly depressed about some event or some end result which you did not want does not mean that the world has come to an end. That's an event, a single event, and not necessarily the totality of your world. Your life goes on even in the event of serious disasters.

Seven: You have to honestly accept your abilities and heartlessly examine your strengths and weaknesses. Some people do better with their hands and some people do better with their heads but in order to do better with your head and to do better with your hands, it is necessary to practice. Very few talents come naturally to a point of perfection. It is very rare that anyone becomes a concert pianist without spending hours on end of hard work devoted to the practice of the piano. The same thing is true of any intellectual or artistic activity even though the spirit and the biological urges which drive those activities is necessary. In order take the initiative there has to be the perseverance and the persistence to practice those skills to such a point they then do become more perfect, and automatic. Thomas Edison is said to have defined inventing: one percent inspiration and ninety-nine percent perspiration.

Eight: Scrutinize your physical assets and liabilities, your appearance, your defects, your body shape, etc. that you may see the positive physical aspects of what you are but also be apprised of the negative, of what you are not. You can not blame yourself if your genetic structure is such that you are endowed with a metabolism which does not lend you to being thin, tall, blue eyes when you would like to have brown eyes; or thick hair when you would like to have thick hair or thin hair where you would like to have thin hair or hair over your entire body and wish it weren't there. These are genetic aberrations which you have to take into account but if you allow them to dominate your feelings about yourself then you are bound to fail because these are not the things that can be changed. What will count will be how you manage yourself with those discrepancies of what is "normal".

What is idealistically normal is a mythical composite of the people who exist with their "abnormalities". Don't forget that the idea that we dream of so far as our figures and our facial configurations are concerned, anatomy and all these features is a composite idea. It is not something that comes to very many people. Only one in hundreds of thousands of people is actually born with an "ideal" appearance. They are born that way. You can improve what you have but to understand it best is to use it to your advantage which really makes the difference. In this sense it is not what you are that makes so much difference, it is what you think about yourself, about what you are and how you manage yourself with those "abnormalities".

Nine: Don't expect everyone else to be perfect. Everyone else's personality is also flawed in some manner and if we wait for the "perfect" person to come along and we will settle for nothing else we are in for a hard, long, lonely, and probably fruitless search.

A professional's awareness of his ignorance is not sufficient knowledge to be able to take the responsibility for attempting to assist other individuals in the reorganization of their lives. The amount of information which is contained in that professional's awareness is minuscule.

A passing acquaintance with what are called social dynamics, or society, is not sufficient information with which to take the responsibility of directing other people in how to live their lives. The physician who does not have any special contact with social knowledge in reference to personal and interpersonal relationships, does not have sufficient knowledge to undertake assisting individuals in examining their lives. However, of all the professionals, the physician is the one who has the most direct responsibility for "life and death" in the manner in which he practices and the way in which he attempts to treat people. That is because it makes no difference what his specialty in medicine is, what he does in ordering medication, surgery or various physical manipulations of a person including possibly the capacity to manipulate the patient's mind by his attitude toward the patient and as well as what he says, is a responsibility which physicians feel strongly because they have the responsibility of life or death. Other professionals do not carry the same load of responsibility as does the physician.

Gradually over the years philosophical attitudes about medical treatment have changed. Traditionally the physician is educated to treat the individual patient for the sake of the patient. A second goal is the treatment of the patient for the sake of society (as in many mental and correctional institutions). A third facet has now occurred politically as well as in the field of public health, ie: the treatment of society for the sake of the individual - as in evidence the political push currently in progress to create a National Medical Insurance Plan which is untested. Of all those National Medical Insurance Plans (Socialized Medicine) which have been put into use around the world all are worse than the Fee for Service plan in the United States. They are much more expensive, render less service, and are much more ponderous in the delivery of services to the individual. They stifle innovation and progress.

The fourth consideration is the alteration of society for the sake of society and that is what communism was all about. It has failed miserably in every respect .

On a daily basis any specialty in medicine, including psychiatry, does have the legal authority and also the responsibility to write prescriptions for you on a planned basis based on a formal diagnosis of what your condition is, whether it be physical or mental.

Even though professionals other than physicians try to attain the depth of the knowledge to which a physician is exposed they are not charged with the responsibility of monitoring life and death even though they are licensed in their particular profession.

The only person, in my opinion, who is educated and charged with the responsibility of caring for the mind as well as the body is the psychiatrist. Other specialties in medicine do not study the effects of the medication on the mind and the central nervous system anywhere near as strenuously as do the psychiatrists.

Psychologists, on the other hand, do make far more specialized study of the interrelationships between individuals and in the consideration of the abstract formulation of what the mind is. Those studies have no specific relationship to the physiological functioning of the mind and now there are specialists, as I have mentioned previously, in psychology who call themselves neuropsychologists and who presumably study the neurophysiology of the mind as well as studying the abstractions which are called mental processes.

Even neuropsychologists do not study the direct affects of drugs and the interactions of drugs of all kinds so they are thereby prohibited from making and giving prescriptions because of their lack of education in that field of knowledge.

The social workers are further limited by the fact that they have a knowledge of society and they study the agencies in society, usually in one particular geographical area, but at the same time their study of the agencies in society prepares them to expand their knowledge if they move from one region or geopolitical area to another and with the knowledge that they have, they can relatively quickly get to know the ins and outs of the various agencies where they might be able to refer you for help. Social workers study group therapy and they feel confident to do group therapy but that is based on premises similar to the psychologists. On the abstractions of the means by which the mind works and the theories of mental functioning which are not based on any neurophysiological theories.

The social worker does have specialized knowledge about types of group or community services which are available and this can be a very distinct help when you are trying to find someone to offer you the opportunity to help yourself when that need arises.

The social worker is not capable of any neurophysiological, medicinal or surgical approaches to affect a change in another person.

Some of the most difficult words in the English language for a professional to learn are "I don't know", "We don't know" or "No one knows".

To accept this lack of knowledge, to not have all the answers, is a very humbling experience for any professional, including physicians and psychiatrists. It takes a great deal of experience and self examination on the part of any professional to accept that conclusion and not try to offer an answer for every conceivable symptom or discomfort which you may have.

The more recent catch word of theoretical structure representing the complexity of the individual as well as social interrelationships is biopsychosocial living. The concept is such that it is difficult or impossible to grasp in it's whole. It implies that people are exposed and react to such elements of the universe, of our biology and of our sociology and culture to integrate in themselves and that is what they are, what they become and where they came from, including the heavens..

Copernicus contributed to the biopsychosocial concept by creating the arithmetic calculus which is often applied to outer space and of course the influence of outer space on mankind is still subject to speculation and is being studied by super specialists, astronomers, physicists, physicians, in a continuous process. The General Systems Theory of Ludwig Von Bertalanffy is a system of thinking about the complexity of systems including man and his relationship with the universe, with each other and with himself. Immanuel Velikovsky is another individual who studied the interrelationships of man with outer space and on the face of the earth itself. As a matter of fact he studied man's relationship with his gods and demonstrated that the various religious texts which exist in the world are actually historical accounts of what occurred during that period of time. He was able to demonstrate by semantic analysis of those texts that the events which happened in the eastern part of the world had a simultaneous opposite corresponding event in the western part of the world.

Immanuel Velikovsky wrote a book in which he tried to write mathematical formulas for each and all of the various chemical processes going on in the human body and was able to make a very significant statement about the complexity of those processes. He was firmly convinced that all biological processes could be expressed as mathematical formulas and he had an intellectual goal to render all such biological, social, galaxial, astronomical processes into mathematical formulas.

What I am saying is that there is no aspect of existence, regardless of how it is expressed, that does not impinge on our lives, directly or indirectly, which is what the concept of the biopsychosocial complex abstraction attempts, to state all in one word.

Regardless of the complexities of these abstractions, fundamentally you are the only one who can mentally examine yourself better than anyone else and I highly recommend that you proceed to try to do that.

The simplest of life's biological functions are shared by everyone and the eating, drinking, the defecation, urination, sexual relations. They are shared because of their universality in all of the biological world. These are the natural functions which exist. To make an opponent of them is to go out of your way to make believe that they don't exist and will only draw attention to yourself negatively. They are natural functions that everybody experiences. They should not have to be either exaggerated nor should they be apologized for; nor should they be exploited as though they were some disadvantage or some major advantage. These are the natural aspects of life over which we have no control insofar as our conscious function is concerned. At best, if we want to change them it takes a major effort and usually the changes that can be accomplished are very minuscule compared with what nature provides us.

Whether we are male or female, each of us needs the other sex if we wish to see ourselves replaced in the world after we have left it and that is an inescapable event. Some of our desires cannot be achieved alone. Children for example cannot be created alone although with current scientific technologies children are sometimes started outside the womb and outside the body. None the less they are still nourished inside the body and the legal battles trying to untangle the complexities of surrogate mothers or surrogate fathers or sperm or ovum banks is increasingly complex. These entanglements and legalities are such that there will always be tremendous arguments about who is what in relation to the offspring.

Define your goals in being alive. You are alive. Define what you feel the cause for your being alive is; define, if you can, what you feel the origin of your being alive is. It makes no difference to me whether you define the origin of your being alive as being theological or evolutionary or explosive or retroactive or implosive. Whatever it is, set yourself the task of thinking about these philosophical questions to decide for yourself what you feel is the right concept for you and what you conclude where you came from or where you are going.

Your satisfactions in what you do to feel satisfaction is one thing but to think about it and how it comes about and how you have achieved that goal is also something. It is necessary, in order for you to get the most out of life, to be able to define as well as experience those satisfactions so that you know how to seek them in whatever capacity it is possible for you to seek them.

Do the same thing with your frustrations. Nobody is pleased with everything or everybody There are people who will not like you for what ever reason and they probably don't know what that reason is. There are also people that you won't like and you may not be able to define why you do not like them for what ever reason. You may seem to feel that they are awesome, fearsome or too self centered, antagonistic towards you or what ever it is. It is not necessary to like everyone but just because you don't like someone doesn't mean that you cannot work with them, that you cannot do some thinking within yourself to smooth out those rough spots and if necessary work with them in spite of adverse feelings.

It is also true that there are people with whom you feel comfortable from the first moment you meet them. It doesn't have to be sexual attraction but you just feel good to be with them, and they with you. It may feel as though you have known each other all your lives even though you are fully aware that you met only "this afternoon".

It is also necessary for you to explore your dissatisfaction with what is going on culturally, politically and economically. You should be able to define for yourself how you fit into those patterns and what thought processes lead you to what you conclude is your business and what you conclude is right for you. What causes trouble is the thought that you can change the world all by yourself. Should you presume to take the action to do so, such as killing off all those people you feel shouldn't exist because they aren't deserving of existence, you are creating more trouble for yourself than you are likely to be able to manage. Society doesn't tolerate that kind of individual control for very long.

Society will tolerate thoughts, concepts and some actions toward making changes in what ever is going on but those changes have to be put in terms of what society has now, as well as how you see it. I'm not trying say that it is necessary for you to agree with everything that's happening but if you try to revolutionize society in one fell swoop then you will be creating trouble for yourself.

There are a lot of realities that are unfair; a lot of interrelationships, restrictions and sometimes favors which are grossly unfair to other members of society as well as to you. Your feelings about that are what is important and how you manage to express those feelings is what becomes most important.

Allow your thoughts to flow freely. What do you have to fear? What is there in the world to be afraid of, really, except ourselves? Life has always been treacherous. Life has always been fearful. There are always people out there who are trying to take advantage of everybody else which has to be taken as a standard. It is not necessary for you to relate to them and it is not necessary for you to impose them physically on others to such an extent that you get yourself into social trouble by thinking you are better than they are. You don't have to take direct action to see that they get "done in". If you take direct action in those respects you are more likely to find yourself in trouble.

It is also true that if you take direct action in trying to improve your own lot by taking from someone else something which they have and for which they may have worked very hard because you are envious of them having it when you do not have it, then you are also in for trouble. That's what laws are all about. It is necessary for us to control our impulses to take those kinds of actions if we are to get along in this world.

If you surpress anything in your thoughts and cut them off as being too unimportant, or too frivolous, or too serious, or too irrelevant, then you are likely to have some problems. You have to set a part of yourself aside methodically to examine yourself thoroughly about what ever thoughts there are that do go through your mind.

It doesn't make any difference how much education you have. It is how you use what you have that makes the difference. Some of the most successful people have not been formally well educated they have been self educated. In a sense all people are self educated. I believe that there is no teaching; there is only learning. There are ways of doing these things which are within the realm of acceptability and to progress but in order to do so it is necessary for you to allow your anxieties to guide you whenever it is desirable to be anxious. There are some situations in which fear is a very appropriate and necessary part of life but on the other hand if you let such fear control you in your actions then you are certainly going to have much more difficulty both in overcoming the fear and in extricating yourself from the situation which caused the fear. It is possible that we may not be individually extricated from the situations which cause the fear.

Death itself is a reality. We don't have to like it and we don't have to think we will enjoy it but it is not something we experience. Death we don't experience. When we're dead we're dead. What we experience is being alive.

When you have goals set up for yourself and you feel you can know yourself better then you have also to take concrete steps to make "stepping stones" toward those goals. If those goals are not as completely achieved as you would like them to be it is necessary to rearrange your goals but you should have long term as well as short term goals. Most of the long term goals are achieved by achieving the short term goals.

There will be some things in your life in which you might achieve as milestones; for example, being born is a milestone in your existence; going through puberty is a milestone in your existence; going through marriage is a milestone in your existence; having children, for both men and women, is a milestone in your existence; death is a milestone in your existence even though death in and of itself terminates your existence nonetheless it is still a milestone; other milestones may be not as advantageous or not as pleasant. Physical injuries and illnesses are all events which may be either stepping stones or milestones depending on the impact which you allow them to have on you.

A major physical illness for example is something you may have no control over, a major burn, may be a milestone in your existence because even though you dislike it and you didn't want it to happen; you wish it never did happen; that doesn't change what did happen. It is necessary to adjust to those circumstances to the best of your ability to do so. If you let those events block you and then you proceed to feel you're no good and depressed and not worthwhile then you are going to be much worse off than you are now. Independence means swim or sink.

Von Bertalanffy, Ludwig
    General Systems Theory (paper)
    Geo. Braziller, N.Y. 1968

    Robots, Men and Minds
    Geo Braziller, N.Y. 1967

Velikovsky, Immanuel
    Worlds in Collision
    1950